ABSTRACT

In early 2014, 3 West African states of Guinea, Liberia, and Sierra Leone made news headlines when Ebola virus disease (EVD) ravaged the sub-region. The Liberian government was ill-equipped to efficiently contain EVD outbreak due to inadequate training for hospitals and health care workers. The government's mandatory cremation policies and the banning of public gatherings significantly contributed to the spread of EVD. EVD infected 10,666 and 4,808 died from the disease in the first 6 months of the epidemic. The purpose of this case study research was to examine the social, economic, and policy factors that contributed to the spread of EVD in the city of Monrovia, Liberia, where one of the largest outbreaks occurred. Using the Bandura Social Cognitive Theory (SCT) as the theoretical framework, in-depth interviews were conducted to explore the phenomenon of 30 participants. The participants included 10 EVD survivors, 10 family caregivers, 2 government officials, 4 nongovernmental organizations staff, 2 academicians, and 2 members from the media. Data were collected through interviews, observations and documentation. Snowball sampling was utilized, and NVivo 10 software was used to code and create themes. The findings show that EVD survivors and family caregivers experienced simultaneous episodes of hoping for their desirable outcomes while at the same time anticipating the worst to happen. This study may positively impact the people of Liberia and the world as a whole by promoting positive social and policy changes. It may provide information for improving future policies and training of healthcare workers and the general public during future EVD outbreaks.

COPING WITH THE THREAT OF EBOLA:
A CASE STUDY

By

Dr. Augustine Manneh Sumo

MBA, University of Phoenix, 2013

MPH, California State University – Fullerton, 2007

BS, University of Liberia, 1994

Dissertation Submitted in Fulfillment

of the Requirements for the Degree of

Doctor of Philosophy

Public Policy and Administration – Law and Public Policy

Walden University

August 2017

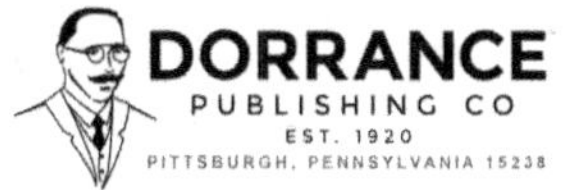

Dorrance Publishing Co
585 Alpha Drive
Pittsburgh, PA 15238
Visit our website at *www.dorrancebookstore.com*

ISBN: 978-1-6491-3316-8
eISBN: 978-1-6491-3283-8

DEDICATION

After being furious with my house-help for not letting me know soon enough to restock our food closet, I walked out of my living room angry and went outside to be alone and not being bother. Efe, my eldest daughter walked over to me and said "daddy you have to do better than this, this is too simple to go under your skin. Remember you are the leader, you are the doctor, so cheer up." "Daddy, you look like a big man in the eyes of many so you have to take that position and don't let anger rob you of your ability to lead" she further lamented. I asked her, where are you coming from with these wise words? She looked me in the eyes and replied. "Don't forget that you always told us to be patient and to handle issues with a peaceful mind and without fear or favor." "Don't forget that you are my doctor and I want everyone in the world to call you Dr. Sumo." You will make a great man in society, she said.

Rebecca Efe Sumo, may your soul rest in peace. You shared only 19 valuable years with us on earth. Today, I am proud that I followed your dream; I am Dr. Augustine Manneh Sumo. I won't have made it here without the love, care, values, and encouragement given to me by you. You believed in me when no one did. You suffered and died from pain while I was away seeking a greener pasture for us. I can imagine your last moment, how you cried and call my name for help, but I was not there to help you. You cried alone. Sleep on, you gentle soul. Daddy loves you. Celebrating this milestone is difficult without you. Therefore, I hereby dedicate this dissertation to you. Your memory and love will forever live in my heart and the hearts of the many you touched. Your usual words of encouragement thus agreed with Daniel Keyes, who in his poem entitled; Flowers for Algernon stated: "How many great men didn't know enough, or have enough faith in the creative process and themselves"? My journey has been challenged with the experiences of enduring "pain" in almost every sphere of life. Losing my 19 year daughter is the worst experience I have to live with. I also dedicate this dissertation to all children around the world who suffered and died from pain. May the pain of every living being be completely cleared away. May I be the doctor and the medicine, and may I be the nurse for all sick beings in the world until everyone is healed (Prayer for world peace by Geshe Acharya Thubten Loden).

ACKNOWLEDGMENTS

I am very grateful to:

Dr. Lori Ann Demeter, the Chair of my dissertation committee, your patience and entertaining encouragement helped me to complete this dissertation journey. Dr. Timothy Fadgen for taking an interest in my topic of study and supporting me with his wisdom and courage. I am also pleased to acknowledge the followings: Dr. Isaac Washington Browne, Joseph Arku Cole, Alex Victor Cummings, Alex Y. Dossen, James S. Kerkula, Georgine Y. Berrian-Massaquoi, Fate Alex Moore, Kervin Piliporlor, Albert B. Seh, Jackson T.S. Seton, Moses D. Sandy, Emma Majay Sumo, Evelyn N. Sumo, Hawa Sumo-Sengbe, Stephenett T. Carr, Felecia Pakie Sumo, Madison Sumo, Femo Roberts, and Leila Sumo. Special acknowledgement to Pastor Brad Martin and the wonderful congregation of Trinity Presbyterian Church in Wilmington, Delaware. Special thanks to James and Phyllis Albert, and all those I cannot mention. During my lifetime, I have met people who added positively to my purpose. To those who may have hurt me, I want to acknowledge you because that, which did not kill me, made me a survivor. I thank each of you for playing a role in the achievement of my Ph.D. To my dear daughter, Rebecca Efe Sumo who is not fortunate to celebrate this milestone, I say Rest in Peace in the Lord. To my beloved wife Mrs. Moira Boakai-Sumo, I have learned that life is not about waiting for the storm to pass. Life is about dancing in the rain. Thanks for believing in me.

TABLE OF CONTENTS

LIST OF TABLES

LIST OF FIGURES

CHAPTER 1

INTRODUCTION TO THE STUDY

Ebola virus disease (EVD) was first heard of in 1976 when the disease simultaneously surfaced in the Democratic Republic of Congo (DRC) and Sudan (Jones, 2011). Since then, several outbreaks of EVD have occurred in other parts of Africa. The 2014 EVD outbreak in West Africa was the largest and most complex of all EVD outbreaks combined (World Health Organization [WHO], 2015). The West African 2014 EVD outbreak began in the Republic of Guinea in late December 2013, and rapidly spread to Sierra Leone and then into Liberia. The city of Monrovia in Liberia became the hardest hit by the 2014 EVD outbreak (WHO, 2015).

In this qualitative research study, I have articulated how residents of Monrovia coped with the threat of EVD. I explored the social, economic, and policy factors that contributed to the spread of the 2014 EVD outbreak in Liberia. I investigated how mandatory cremation and government's regulations intended to contain the virus further contributed to the spread of EVD. I also explored how Monrovians perceived EVD and what their reactions were towards persons affected by EVD. I further explicated the public's perception and change in attitudes and the meanings they ascribe to EVD. I conducted the study in Monrovia, the capital city of Liberia in West Africa, where one of the 2014 EVD outbreaks occurred. Monrovia was hardest hit by the 2014 EVD outbreak because most Liberians depend on the city for trade and jobs, thus creating a fluid population movement across the country which may have exposed the city to the high rate of EVD transmission and mortality (Chan, 2014).

Most studies continue to focus largely on the poverty and cultural factors for spreading the virus (Chowell & Nishiura, 2014; Tambo, 2014; Tosh &

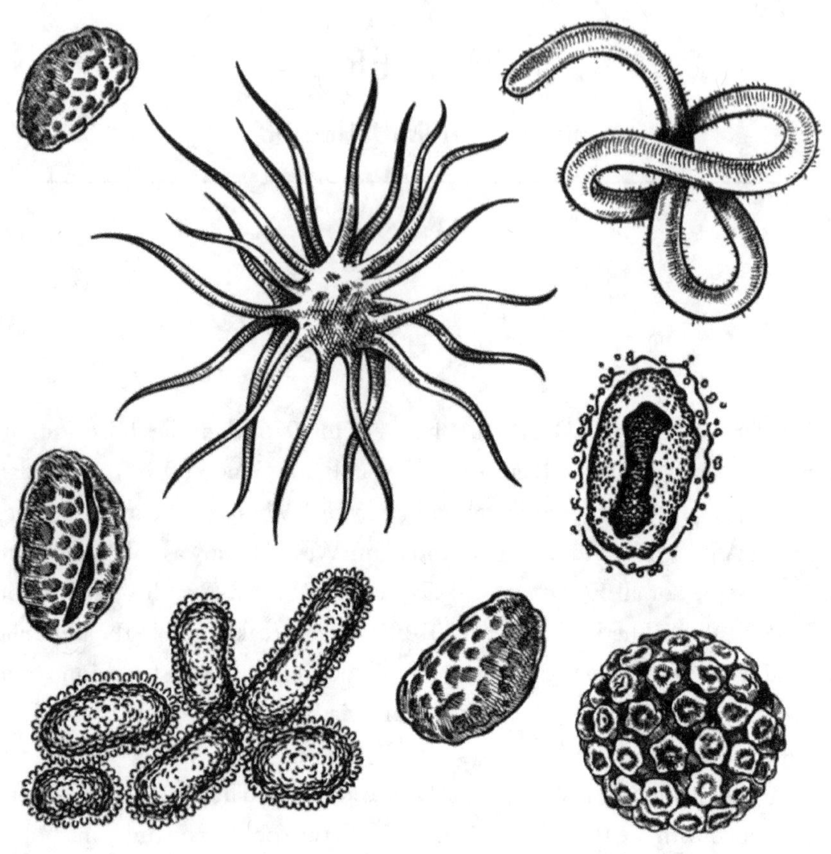

Ebola Virus Disease

Ebola virus disease is also known as Ebola haemorrhagic fever. Studies have shown that it is an emerging zoonotic disease. Ebola is a severe and contagious disease affecting humans and non-human primates.

Ebola kills about 90 % of those infected, but patients have a better chance of survival if they receive early diagnosis and treatment. The virus for now has no cure, or vaccine. The disease first emerged in 1976 in the Democratic Republic of Congo and Sudan. The infection is named after the Ebola River located in Yambuku, Democratic Republic of Congo.

Courtesy of ole.int

Sampathkumar, 2014). With this background, I conducted the study. I have underscored the need to understand what it takes to cope with the threat of EVD and how government's decree and regulations intended to contain the virus may have also influenced the spread of EVD. The main motivation for this study was to articulate the public's perceptions about EVD, which stem from the need to understand what social, policy, and economic factors may have contributed to the spread of EVD. I accomplished these goals by conducting a case study using a qualitative approach.

This dissertation is organized into five chapters: Chapter 1 introduced the study with a historical background and followed by the statement of the problem; the purpose of the study; the nature of the study; the social significance; research questions and the theoretical framework; scope of the study; and assumption, limitations, and delimitations. Chapter 2 is composed of the review of related literature to include the theoretical framework, data collection strategies, factors for the transmission and spread of EVD, the role of the media during epidemics, the role of government and community reaction to EVD, and current healthcare and policy initiatives. In Chapter 3, I described the research design and methodology employed for this study, including the role of the researcher, sample size, instruments, data analysis plan, trustworthiness, and ethical procedures. In Chapter 4, I focused primarily on the results of the study. Chapter 4 also discussed the setting of the study, research questions, demographics, data collection, data analysis, and evidence of trustworthiness. Finally, Chapter 5 included the interpretation of the findings, limitations of the study, recommendations, and implication for social change.

I designed this research to explicate and understand the experiences of EVD survivors, family caregivers, nongovernmental organization (NGO) staff, academicians, and reporters from the media and governmental policy aspects of containing EVD. I underscored the need for policy makers, health care providers, and the general public to understand how people coped with the threat of EVD; including how they perceived EVD; what their reactions symbolized, and what the experience means to them. Chowell and Nishiura (2014) argued that articulating such lived experiences helps generate information that may be used to explain people's reactions during outbreaks and can also be useful in enabling health caregivers and policy makers to better prepare the population for future outbreaks.

I relied primarily on the inputs from selected EVD survivors and their family caregivers who experienced the 2014 EVD outbreak in three selected communities in Monrovia. I also solicited inputs from governmental policy makers from the Ministry of Health and Social Welfare and nongovernmental organizations (NGOs) such as Médecins Sans Frontières (MSF) and the Liberia National Red Cross (LNRC) who provided care for the 2014 EVD survivors. I further solicited inputs from academicians and reporters from the media.

Data were collected through interviews, observations, and documentation. For this study, I selected 30 participants in three communities that were the hardest hit by the 2014 EVD in Monrovia. I anticipated that at least 10 of the 30 research participants were EVD survivors and 10 family caregivers in each of the three communities; whereas the other 10 participants included government officials, NGO staff, academicians, and reporters from the media. These survivors and their family caregivers including NGO staff, academicians, and reporters from the media experienced the phenomenon and can better explain how they coped with the threat of EVD.

Because Liberians, in general, share a lot in common such as culture and tradition, it was assumed that individuals in the three selected communities can reflect the identity of the entire city of Monrovia. According to Bellizzi (2014), addressing such real-life experiences reinforces community health education campaigns, which serves to reduce the widespread fear, panic, and hysteria that characterizes an EVD epidemic.

Bellizzi (2014) explained that during the 1976 EVD outbreaks in Sudan and the Democratic Republic of Congo (DRC), health care workers used three main interventions techniques; coordination, isolation, and treatment to contain the spread of EVD. Bellizzi (2014) further stressed the need for coordination between isolation and treatment as means to contain EVD globally.

BACKGROUND OF THE STUDY

EVD was first identified in 1976 when the virus surfaced in Nzara, Sudan, and in Yambuku, the DRC. The latter outbreak occurred in a village in the DRC near the Ebola River, from which the virus got its name (Jones, 2011). WHO

(2014) explained that since the initial outbreaks of EVD in the DRC and Sudan in 1976, several known EVD outbreaks have occurred in Uganda, Gabon, Italy, the United Kingdom, the United States of America, Nigeria, Senegal, Mali, Spain, and the most recent 2014 West Africa EVD outbreaks in Guinea, Liberia, and Sierra Leone. The 2014 West Africa EVD outbreak is the largest and most complex of all outbreaks combined (WHO, 2015). Diagnosing EVD is a difficult task (Jones, 2011) especially in low-quality health care systems such as in Guinea, Liberia, and Sierra Leone. Guinea, Liberia and Sierra Leone are among the poorest countries in the world (WHO, 2015). Diseases such as malaria, typhoid fever, and meningitis have symptoms similar to those of EVD which makes it difficult to distinguish at an early stage in low-quality resource health systems.

In this section, I informed the reader about the main issues underpinning the study, specifically issues related to the 2014 EVD outbreak in Monrovia. I have aimed to facilitate a better understanding of the social, economic, and policy factors; coupled with the public's perception and beliefs related to the meaning of EVD. I discussed the geographic and demographic details of the study area followed by highlights of cultural beliefs and practices associated with EVD. In addition, I presented the nature of EVD epidemics in Africa followed by highlights of EVD infections in Liberia.

On March 30th, 2014 the first two EVD cases were reported in the Foya district of Lofa County, Liberia. Lofa County is located in Northern Liberia bordering the Republic of Guinea. Foya district is 360 KM by road from Monrovia. The city of Monrovia is 35.52 km² with a population of over 1 million people. According to the Liberia Institute of Statistics and Geo-Information Services (LISGIS, 2014), Monrovia is the political capital of Liberia and it is built on Cape Mesurado along the Atlantic coast in Montserrado County. Monrovia was hardest hit by the 2014 EVD outbreak recording more than 60% of all EVD cases and mortality in the country (WHO, 2015).

The 2014 EVD outbreak negatively affected the city through the canceling of flights, the closing of schools, hospitals, and businesses. Some foreign investors, visitors, and residents left the city for fear of contracting EVD (Chan, 2014; WHO, 2015). EVD has posed a global challenge with no answer in sight for cure and control (WHO, 2015). The 2014 EVD outbreaks that began in Guinea and rapidly spread into neighboring Sierra Leone and then to Liberia has devastated the lives of many including infants, children, and adults. The 2014 EVD outbreak is the largest and most complex of all, that affected people not only in West Africa but other parts of the world including Europe and the United States. EVD outbreaks in West Africa have recorded more cases and deaths than all other previous outbreaks combined (WHO, 2015).

FOYA DISTRICT IN LOFA COUNTY

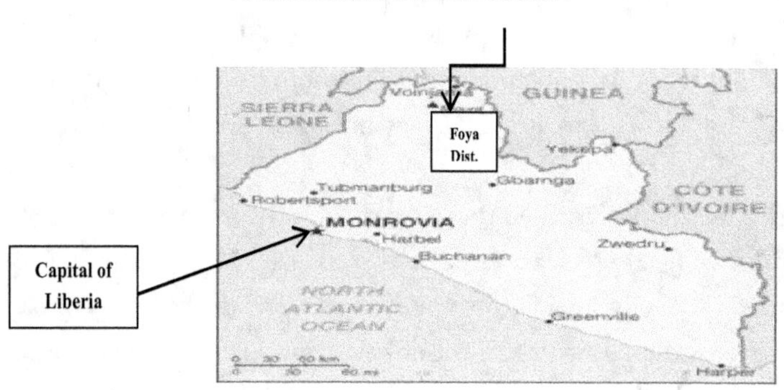

Cases contracted in Liberia............................…....10,666 (as of August 2015)
Deaths...…...4,808 (as of August 2015)
Figure 1. Map of Liberia showing the city of Monrovia and the Foya District in Lofa County, 2015. Source: https://www.google.com/?gws_rd=ssl#q=+ mapof+liberia.

In economic terms, records from LISGIS (2014) indicate that the people of the Foya district in Lofa County heavily depend on agriculture for the production of cash crops and food. LISGIS (2014) further asserted that most farmers of the district trade their goods into neighboring Guinea; where the first EVD outbreak in West Africa was reported in December 2013. The Foya district is predominantly rural, suggesting that most of the populations depend heavily on the forest and forest animals for food and clothing thus implying a regular human-to-animal interaction. According to Tosh and Sampathkumar (2014) and WHO (2015), the human-to-animal contact has been linked to the introduction of EVD infections into human populations from animal natural reservoirs in past outbreaks in the DRC and Sudan.

EVD is known to be among the most virulent pathogens that infect humans and non-humans primates. Early symptoms of EVD include fever, headache, body aches, cough, stomach pain, vomiting, and diarrhea and death within days (Leroy, Gonzalez & Baize, 2011). There are currently five known species of EVD, (a) Bundibugyo Ebolavirus (BEBOV), (b) Zaire Ebolavirus (ZEBOV), and (c) Sudan Ebolavirus (SEBOV), (d) Reston Ebolavirus (REBOV), and (e) Tai Forest Virus (TAVF) formerly known as the Cote d'Ivoire Ebolavirus (CIEBOV). These species of EVD were named after the country where the virus was first isolated (Leroy et al., 2011). Unlike the other four species of EVD, the REBOV does not cause any fatality in humans; however, it is lethal to primates (CDC, 2014; Leroy et al., 2011).

Typically, EVD is a zoonotic disease that can be transmitted to humans through direct contact with live or dead animals that have been infected from a natural reservoir. Currently, the natural reservoir from which EVD is spread into animals is still unknown (Leroy et al., 2011). Feldmann and Geisbert (2012) explained that once the virus enters the human populations, it is spread from person to person through direct contact with the infected blood, fluids, sweat, saliva and semen, and inoculation from contaminated instruments or any contact with infected medical instruments. The potential for human-to-human transmission including high case fatality rate and the lack of defined control mechanism and cure makes EVD a major public health issue globally (WHO, 2015).

Persons infected by EVD would begin to show signs of multiple organ failures by the end of the first 2 weeks of infection. These signs of organ failure according to Feldmann and Geisbert (2012) mean that the patients' condition is worsening and he or she may likely not recover. WHO (2015) explained that during the first week of infection, susceptible patients could experience rapid and extensive viral replication that leads to cell and tissue death in the liver, spleen, lymph nodes, kidney, lung, blood and the gonads. Feldmann and Geisbert (2012) further asserted that these EVD patients will then begin to suffer from a severe headache, sore throat, muscle aches and weakness, and hiccups during the first week. By the second week, patients will begin to vomit and experience severe abdominal pain, followed by diarrhea, pharyngitis, conjunctivitis, multiple organ destruction, and hypovolemic shock, bleeding, and death.

On the other hand, as explained by Feldmann and Geisbert (2012), non-susceptible patients into their second week will begin to show signs of recovery

Symptoms of
Ebola

Headache

Red Eyes

Pharynx and lungs
- Hiccups
- Sore throat
- Difficulty breathing
- Difficulty swallowing

Systemic
- Fever
- Lack of appetite
- Internal bleeding

Chest pain

Muscular
- Aches
- Weakness

Stomach
- Pain
- Vomiting

Joints
- Aches

Skin
- Rash
- Bleeding

Intestines
- Diarrhea

Reservoir and Transmission of Ebola Virus Disease

Ebola is a lethal infection caused by the Ebola virus. It symptoms typically start 2 to 21 days after contracting the virus. The symptoms includes; fever, sore throat and muscle pains, and headaches. It is then followed by nausea, vomiting and diarrhea along with decreased functioning of the liver and kidney, which eventually leads to bleeding. The disease is usually acquired when a person comes into contact with the blood or bodily fluids of an infected animal or person. It is believed that monkeys or fruit bats are the carrier of Ebola virus. However, the main reservoir remains unknown despite many studies.

Courtesy of wikiwand.com

which WHO (2015) asserted are due to the patients' capacity to develop sufficient immunologic response against EVD. WHO (2015) also noted that EVD patients recover slowly, and their recovery is associated with severe wasting, anorexia, amnesia, sexual weakness, visual and hearing difficulties, fatigue, and mental issues. In addition, WHO (2015) explained that EVD survivors may experience episodes of uveitis, ocular pain, photophobia, and increased lacrimation, myalgia, headache, bulimia, sexual weakness, orchitis and amenorrhea, and menstrual disturbances lasting up to 12 months in some survivors.

PSYCHO-SOCIAL CONSEQUENCES OF EBOLA VIRUS DISEASE OUTBREAKS

Normally, when news of EVD outbreaks hit the general public, it becomes a source of psychological and social strain frequently driven by fear (De Roo et al., 1995), inducing news headlines in local, national, and the international press. Since the initial outbreaks of EVD in 1976, news about EVD has continued to create fear and anxiety, leading to far-reaching psychosocial implications on the public even far away from the epicentres of the epidemic (De Roo et al., 1995). WHO (2015) notes that panic gripped Monrovians when EVD killed more than 4,000 patients in less than 6 months. Jerving (2014) described how scary pictures of infected EVD patients and dead bodies being carried from homes on a daily basis triggered widespread fear in the population.

The fear of being infected by neighbors made people to turn away from helping their friends and relatives (WHO, 2015). Those who brave the situation were involved in helping their friends and relatives and as Jerving (2014) noted, they too soon became patients, which further caused fear and panic. For this reason, some communities formed vigilante groups for the purpose of protecting their communities against suspected sources of infection such as EVD survivors, orphans, and health workers (Jerving, 2014). WHO (2015) confirmed that in the process of protecting their communities from the spread of EVD, vigilante groups vandalized and destroyed survivors' properties including quarantining centers.

CULTURAL CLASSIFICATION, BELIEFS, AND PRACTICES RELATED TO EBOLA VIRUS DISEASE

In Monrovia and Liberia as a whole, the concept of virus or disease and illness, in general, is frequently associated with the world of spirits. Hewlett and Amola (2003) argued that these spirits which are believed to be either 'good' or 'bad' affect human lives in both good and bad ways. That is, the good spirits are believed to protect humans against harm, misfortune or disease; whereas the bad spirits would inflict disease, misfortune or suffering. This belief system is structured around the notion that protection from the spirits is directed at individuals who respect social, cultural and religious rituals and practices. West Africans believe that individuals or families who abandon the norms of the good spirits risk being turned over to the bad spirits for punishment. The same applies to the 2014 EVD outbreaks in West Africa and Liberia in particular. In Monrovia, most residents believed that EVD was a result of a curse placed on the people by their gods for wrong doings. Some people in Liberia specifically residents of Monrovia also believe that the EVD outbreak was a hoax designed by the Liberian government to get money from the international community (Jerving, 2014).

Therefore, understanding of the social, economic, and policy factors and peoples' experiences, especially the impact of government's regulations and how residents of Monrovia coped with the threat of EVD; coupled with the deep-seated beliefs about EVD is foundational to designing appropriate epidemic response plans that address the human side of future epidemics. WHO (2015) affirmed that such response plan is particularly important given Liberia's vulnerability to future outbreaks due to the country's low quality health system.

Several scholarly works served as the key foundational literature that relates to EVD. Bellizzi (2014) described the three main interventions used to contain EVD outbreaks in 1976 and recommended the need for coordination between isolation and treatment. Chan (2014) pointed out that although there might be psychological or cultural factors that influenced the spread of EVD, poverty plays a significant role in the spread of the virus. Chowell and Nishiura (2014) stated that the lack of public health infrastructures and control measures at health care centers in Guinea, Liberia, and Sierra Leone caused the spread of the virus. De Roo et al. (1995) stated that denial and fears are the main feelings for EVD survivors, and believing in God was their source of hope for survival.

Gomes et al. (2014) argued that due to the poor health infrastructures of the affected West African countries, and coupled with the global challenge of finding a cure or appropriate preventative measures for EVD, the disease is far from containment. On the other hand, Hodge, Barraza, Measer, and Agrawal (2014) argued that even though cultural factors might have influenced the spread

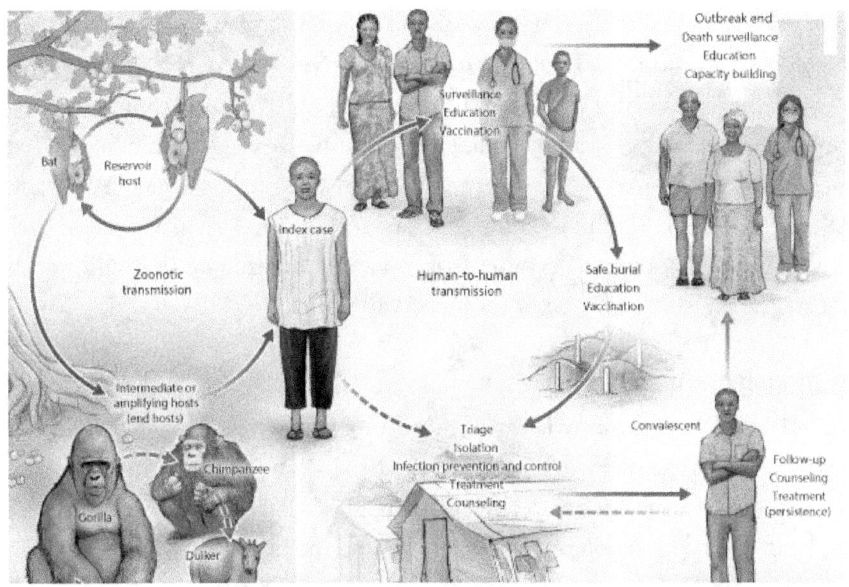

Reservoir and Transmission of Ebola Virus Disease

Fruit bats and other wild animals are believed to carry and spread the virus without being affected by it. Once infection of a human occurs, the disease may be spread from one person to another. Ebola kills about 90 % of those infected, but patients have a better chance of survival if they receive early diagnosis and treatment. The virus for now has no cure, or vaccine. The disease first emerged in 1976 in the Democratic Republic of Congo and Sudan. The infection is named after the Ebola River located in Yambuku, Democratic Republic of Congo.

Courtesy of New England Journal of Medicine

of EVD, poverty and public transportation played a major role in the spread of EVD in Guinea, Liberia, and Sierra Leone. They warned that EVD could reach across the globe if effective control measures are not implemented. Lamontagne et al. (2014) researched the beliefs in God versus clinical intervention and found that the lack of resources and supportive care for EVD patients led to the high incidence of mortality. Tambo (2014) argued that poverty is a driving force behind the spread of EVD. Tosh and Sampathkumar (2014) explored traditional practices (use of animal skins for costumes, eating bush meat, burial rites) that contributed to the spread of EVD in West Africa. Jones (2011) and WHO (2014; 2015) examined those behavioral practices such as funeral rites (cultural beliefs), poverty, economic factors, and hunting and eating of bush meat that caused the spread of EVD in West Africa.

STATEMENT OF THE PROBLEM

In 2014 the city of Monrovia experienced an EVD outbreak, characterized by widespread panic, ostracism, and social stigma. Ramifications of inadequate governmental response to contain the spread of EVD further escalated fear and panic. The infection of 10,666 persons and the deaths of 4,808 patients in six months raised the need for global concern and intervention (Chan, 2014; WHO, 2015). WHO (2015) attests that 375 health workers were infected, and 189 of them died. Monrovia became the hardest hit recording more than 60% of the overall EVD mortality in Liberia (WHO, 2015). Government actions such as mandatory cremation and the banning of public gatherings intended to contain the spread of EVD proved futile thus exacerbating the situation. Monrovians adamantly opposed the cremation and public gatherings policies (regulations) claiming that these violated their traditional ancestral burial rites. These actions further complicated the containment of EVD (Chan, 2014). According to Tosh and Sampathkumar (2014), hygiene rules and safety measures such as avoiding handshake, washing of hands, funeral rites, and the wearing of appropriate personal protective equipment (PPE) by health workers intended to contain the spread of EVD were ignored or lacking.

Liberians, in general, depend on the city of Monrovia for trade and jobs, thus causing a fluid population movement throughout the country. The banning of public gatherings during the EVD outbreak further complicated the situation as residents were seen violating such restrictions (Bellizzi, 2014). On the other hand, the violation of public gatherings or movement during the EVD outbreak may have exposed the city to the high rate of EVD infection and mortality (Chan, 2014). In a recent study, Bellizzi (2014) described the three primary interventions techniques such as coordination, isolation and treatment, and contact tracings and follow-ups. These techniques were effectively used to contain past EVD outbreaks in 1976 when the virus first appeared in Sudan and the DRC. Most studies continue to focus largely on the poverty, economic and social-cultural factors for spreading EVD, thereby underscoring the need to understand what it takes to cope with the threat of EVD including the stigma EVD affected on survivors, the community reactions to EVD survivors, and the effect of governmental laws and policies.

I designed this study to fill in a gap by understanding what it takes to cope with the threat of EVD including the stigma EVD impacted on survivors, community reactions to EVD survivors, and the effect of governmental laws and policies. In this vein, a case study research using a qualitative approach was designed and applied. This research was intended to explicate and understand the experiences of EVD survivors, family caregivers, academicians, and reporters from the media, governmental and nongovernmental organizations (NGOs) policy aspects of containing EVD. This means that it is still unclear how people cope with the threat of EVD and its social stigma, including how they perceive the virus, what their reactions symbolize and what the experience means to them. Literature continues to explain the poverty, economic and social-cultural factors for spreading EVD, but there is no clear or existing literature to explain what it takes to cope with the threat of EVD including its social stigma, community reactions and the effect of governmental laws and policies during an EVD outbreak.

PURPOSE OF THE STUDY

The purpose of this qualitative case study was to explore the social, economic and policy factors that contributed to the spread of the 2014 EVD outbreak in Liberia. This study utilized a case study methodology that falls within Yin's (2014) qualitative case study research tradition. Studies have indicated that poverty and culture lifestyles influenced the spread of the 2014 EVD (Chan, 2014; Tosh & Sampathkumar, 2014). To understand how poverty and culture lifestyles influenced the spread of the 2014 EVD, this study relied on the inputs from EVD survivors, their family caregivers, officials of government, NGO staff, academicians, and reporters from the media who directly or indirectly experience EVD. Specifically, this study was designed to gain a clear understanding of how people experienced the phenomenon of coping with the threat of EVD; especially, how they perceived EVD and the change in attitudes of survivors, what their reactions towards EVD symbolized, including their reactions towards persons and families affected by EVD. Additionally, the study explored how governments' decrees and regulations further influenced the spread of EVD instead of containing it. In economic terms, the study investigated how petty trading contributed to the spread of the EVD.

RESEARCH QUESTIONS

The research questions for this study focused on the phenomenon of coping with the threat of EVD, including the social, cultural and economic factors, social stigma and governmental policies. They were:

RQ1: How did survivors and family caregivers cope with the threat of EVD in Monrovia in 2014?

RQ2: What social, cultural, and economic factors may have contributed to the spread of EVD in Monrovia in 2014?

RQ3: How did government policies of mandatory cremation and banning of public gatherings affect the containment of EVD in Monrovia in 2014?

RQ4: What social stigma did EVD cause among survivors?

THEORETICAL FRAMEWORK

The theoretical base for this study was the Social Cognitive Theory (SCT) which was originally developed by Miller and Dollard in 1941. Later, Bandura and Walters advanced the theory in 1963 with the principles of observational learning and vicarious reinforcement. By 1986, the SCT had fully developed, positing that learning can occur in social context with a dynamic and reciprocal interaction of the person, the environment, and behavior. The SCT emphasizes social influence on external and internal social reinforcements such as determining learning and subsequently behavior.

The SCT explained the manner in which an individual can acquire and maintain a certain behavior, as well as taking into consideration the social environment where the individual may perform the behavior. The SCT provided strategies for intervention to include an evaluation model based on environmental factors. The SCT also provided a framework for designing and implementing programs (Bandura, 1997). The SCT is unique for this study because; it dealt with the cognitive and emotional aspects of a person. It also dealt with the behavioral aspects of understanding a behavioral change in a person. Second, the SCT provided opportunities for future behavioral research when a study leaves gaps that need to be studied, and it allows for other theoretical frameworks to provide new insights and understanding (Bandura, 1997). According to Bandura (1997), environment influenced the individual, and the individual influences the environment.

Furthermore, Miller and Morris (2014) outlined three basic concepts in the SCT: (a) that people can learn through observation and emulate those observed behaviors, (b) inner psychological states are a critical part of the education process, and (c) an individual skill acquisition does not necessarily equate to a change in behavior. Human self-regulatory capability plays the central role in SCT, as it does in other prominent theories of self-regulation and motivation (Stajkovic & Luthans, 1998b). Deci and Ryan (2002) argued that self-regulation is the highest level of learning which allows individuals to adjust their learning strategies to contextual and personal changes. In this regard, individuals may be able to start using strategies to adapt themselves to contextual and circumstantial characteristics and be motivated by self-efficacy perceptions of potential situations.

On the other hand, Bandura (1997) stated that self-efficacy belief serves as an important motivational source driven by an individual's judgment about his or her abilities to organize and perform some actions to achieve desirable goals and functions. Coping under the threat of EVD relates to the above argument as EVD survivors may have been stigmatized as a result of EVD. Dee Roo et al. (1995) used the social representation theory (SRT) to explore the behavior of EVD survivors in Kibale, Uganda upon initially hearing that they have survived from EVD and declared Ebola-free. Due to the constant challenges of coping with the threat and physical symptoms of EVD, survivors graced the news with distrust. The label "survivor" has stigmatized them and the news was received with cautiousness and hesitation. Helman (2007) explained that in situations such as EVD outbreaks, people respond differently, some will turn to their natural environment, and others will turn to supernatural forces for cure or healing. Helman (2007) noted that because of the great importance culture plays in ones live; it is crucial to understand the socio-cultural dimensions underlying people's health values, beliefs, and behaviors. The SCT subscribed to Helman's (2007) argument affirming that the environment can influence the individual, and the individual influences the environment (Bandura, 1997).

According to the SCT, people may set higher standards for themselves and activate future behaviors to satisfy the new standards (Bandura, 1997). The self-reflective capability in SCT can be defined as human self-reflective consciousness. Self-reflective consciousness enables people to think and analyze their experiences and thought processes. By reflecting on their different personal experiences, participants, health caregivers, and policy makers can generate knowledge about their environment and themselves. More details for the theoretical framework are highlighted in Chapter 2.

NATURE OF THE STUDY

For this research study, a qualitative case study design was used to interview EVD survivors, family caregivers, and officials of government, NGO staff, academicians, and reporters from the media who directly or indirectly experienced the 2014 EVD. I examined the experiences of survivors and their family caregivers including the policy factors regarding the outbreak. The research site was three communities in the city of Monrovia that were the hardest hit by EVD. Permission was granted from the Walden University's IRB to conduct this study. I recruited 30 participants from three communities to conduct data collection. I planned interviews to continue until data saturation was achieved, and I attained this goal with the original 30 participants. I fully explained the nature of the study to the participants, and I also asked the participants to read, understand, and sign an informed consent form to participate in the study. Those who signed and returned the consent forms were allowed to participate in the study.

RESEARCH DESIGN AND METHOD

Yin (2014) defined *research design* as the researchers' comprehensive plan for answering the research questions, which includes strategies to enhance integrity for the study. Such a plan as explained by Yin (2014) should incorporate the researcher's philosophy, strategies of inquiry and a specific method. For this study, I selected a qualitative research design in agreement with Yin's (2014) exposition which is best suited to investigate the experiences of individuals who survived the recent 2014 EVD outbreak in Monrovia. Research method (Yin, 2014) includes specific steps, procedures, and strategies used to collect and analyze the data generated to support the study.

I selected a case study approach for this study because it fits well within the qualitative research domain to investigate coping with the threat of EVD. In the context of a case study approach, McMillian and Schumacher (2001) argued that Yin's theory can support the study by providing multiple sources of evidence. This can be achieved through in-depth interviews, observations, and documentation (triangulation). In this regard, converging lines of inquiry are built thereby ensuring validity and, at the same time, maintaining a chain of evidence. Before choosing an appropriate research design, Yin (2014) advised that researchers should select an approach that incorporates philosophical worldviews, and then identify the approach of inquiry related to the worldview and specific methods of research that translate the approach into real practice. Generally, a qualitative research approach enables the researcher to discover, understand, and describe meanings people assign to their lived experiences.

I selected a case study design in the context of Yin (2014) for this study. With this case study design, I was able to conduct analysis, interpret the research findings, and answer the research questions. Yazan (2015) added that a qualitative inquiry elucidates and entails in-depth and holistic investigation of human phenomena through the collection of rich descriptive data and then analyzing it. In this direction, I continue to sample participants until data saturation was achieved. I collected data from EVD survivors, family caregivers, government officials, NGO staff, academicians, and reporters from the media in three communities that were the hardest hit by EVD in Monrovia. I observed the participants and took notes during the observation process. I solicited documents such as diaries of survivors' and their family caregivers' accounts and experiences about EVD. Participants underwent in-depth interviews that I tape-recorded, digitized and transcribed. I analyzed the data by listening and reviewing the interviews. I obtained and stored data in the following formats; paper (journal), electronic (computer), or audio (tape-recorder). All data were protected using a locked file cabinet for papers and a password protected computer and flash drive (thumb). I ensured full security precautions such as locked cabinets, computer or flash password protection.

Yin (2014) stated that in a case study research, purposeful selection should include participants who have directly or indirectly experienced the phenomenon. It is in this context that other members of the communities who were not infected by EVD were also recruited to inquire their inputs. The participants were passionately interested in understanding the nature and meanings of the phenomenon. Participants were willing to partake in lengthy interviews to include follow-up interviews. I was granted permission (consent) to tape-record the interviews and to publish the data in a dissertation and other publications. Details for this research design and method was discussed in Chapter 3 of this dissertation.

DEFINITIONS OF KEY TERMS

The terms below were relevant to this study:

Coping: The amount of cognitive and behavioral endeavors, which are continually changing, aiming to handle a particular demand, be it internal or external. (Lazarus & Folkman, 1980, p. 223).

Culture: Damen (1987) defined culture as the shared patterns of behaviors and interaction, cognitive constructs, and affective understanding that are learned through a process of socialization. These shared patterns would identify and distinguish members of a culture group (p. 367).

Ebola: Feldmann and Geisbert (2012) described Ebola as an infectious and generally fatal disease characterized by fever and severe internal bleeding. The disease is transmitted through direct human-to-animal contact and spread through human-to-human contact through an infected person (para. 97).

Family-caregiver: A person providing any type of care of physical and or emotional care for an ill or disabled relative at home (Chan, 2014, p. 5).

Fear: In a situation such as epidemic, WHO (2014) defined fear as an emotion caused by the belief that something is dangerous and has the potential to cause pain and threat. People in West Africa and other parts of the world were subjected to fear as EVD ravaged their communities (para. 11).

Liberia: Officially called the Republic of Liberia, Liberia was founded in 1822 by freed slaves from the United States of America and the Caribbean. Liberia is located in West Africa and is bordered by Guinea in the North, Ivory Coast in the East, Sierra Leone in the West, and the Atlantic Ocean on the South. Liberia was the hardest hit by the 2014 EVD outbreak (LIS-GIS, 2014, p. 17).

Monrovia: The capital and the largest city of Liberia in West Africa. The city was named after President James Monroe of the United States. Monrovia was the hardest hit by the 2014 EVD outbreak. The city recorded more than 60% overall for all places where the outbreak occurred (LIS-GIS, 2014, p. 18).

Stigma: A traumatized situation marked with disgrace associated with the quality and value of a person. People or communities associated with any form of stigma such as EVD suffer from social rejection, violence, and diminished quality of life (De Roo et al., 1995, p. 62).

Survivor: WHO (2015) referred to the 2014 EVD survivor as an individual who survived, especially a person who remain alive after a deadly epidemic such as EVD in which many others died. The 2014 EVD outbreak in Monrovia killed over 4,000 people in less than six months (para. 5).

Threat: A person or a disease likely to cause damage or death. In 2014, the EVD outbreak was a major threat to the people of West Africa (De Roo et al., 1995, p. 62).

ASSUMPTIONS

In the course of this study, it was assumed that participants could come up with more information that explains how they coped with the threat of EVD and change in behavior (stigma). It was also assumed that while interviewing participants, new theories or findings and interpretations may emerge that could illustrate or modify existing theories. Since most Liberians share a lot in common such as cultural and traditional practices, it was further assumed that individuals in the three communities could reflect the demographic characteristics and experiences with the outbreak of the entire city of Monrovia. The new information may allow for health caregivers, policymakers, and national governments to solve complex problems in a diverse global community.

SCOPE AND DELIMITATIONS

As stated earlier, Monrovians experienced an EVD outbreak in 2014 that was characterized by widespread panic, ostracism, and social stigma. Consequences of inadequate governmental response to contain the spread of EVD further escalated fear and panic. In 6 months, 10,666 persons were infected by EVD in Liberia, and 4,808 of those infected died. Monrovia became the hardest hit recording more than 60% of the overall EVD mortality in Liberia. I designed this study to understand how Monrovians coped with the threat of EVD including the stigma EVD affected on survivors. I also examined the community reactions to EVD survivors, and the impact of governmental laws and policies during the outbreak. I used a qualitative approach to explicate and understand the experiences of EVD survivors, family caregivers, government officials, NGO staff, academicians, and reporters from the media who directly or indirectly experienced EVD. The SCT was used to explain the manner in which an individual can acquire and maintain a particular behavior. This study was delimited to residents of Monrovia who directly or indirectly experienced the 2014 EVD outbreak.

In order to guarantee the right respondents, I based sampling on the requirements that participants must first be an EVD survivor or a family caregiver still living in the selected community. Or government officials who made policy decisions or NGO staff who provided treatment and isolation, or academicians who witnessed the epidemic, and or reporters from the media who covered the outbreak. In 2015, arrangements to release basic information such as names and contacts of EVD survivors and their family caregivers were concluded with relevant government and nongovernmental institutions that provided care and other services for the 2014 EVD patients in Liberia. These institutions include the Ministry of Health and Social Welfare (MOH&SW) of Liberia, Médecins Sans Frontières (MSF), and the Liberia National Red Cross (LNRC). Upon IRB approval, I sent invitations to EVD survivors and their family caregivers who were identified by the above institutions to voluntarily participate in the study. Invitations were also extended to government officials from the MOH&SW, and NGO staff from MSF and LNRC, including academicians from the communities and reporters from the media who covered the 2014 EVD outbreak to participate in the study.

Transferability addresses the degree to which research can be generalized or transferred to other settings. For this study, transferability was enhanced by closely working on the description of the research framework and by addressing the assumptions that was central to the study (Trochim, 2006). Yin (2014) stated that the representation of samples is not a determinant of transferability in qualitative research, it depends on how well the study allow for the reader to deduce whether similar processes and methods will relate to their own settings. To attain the utmost transferability, it was crucial that I ask the correct questions during interviews.

LIMITATIONS

I used a small sample size of 30 participants comprising EVD survivors, family caregivers, government officials, NGO staff, academicians, and reporters from the media for interviews, observations, and documentation. However, Yin (2014) asserted that the study could be criticized on grounds that the experiences of small numbers of selected research participants cannot be widely generalized for a large group of people. Limitations of this study may be due to the responses of participants that could be skewed due to respondents' bias.

Data for this study primarily depended on interviews which were self-reported. Self-reporting is not always reliable because an individual may provide an answer he or she thinks is correct as opposed to what he or she genuinely feels (Howard, 1980). This bias could diminish the validity of the data. To address this limitation, the interview questions were carefully crafted in order to eliminate or minimize biased responses. Qualitative research is an interpretative research which incorporates personal values, biases, and judgments. Yin (2014) suggests that the researcher's openness should be considered to guide the study so as to make it useful and positive. Another potential limitation to this study was time. I explored all avenues to ensure that more time was available for interviews, observations, and documentation of participants.

SIGNIFICANCE OF THE STUDY

I designed this study to fill in a gap in the scholarly literature by understanding the social, economic, and policy-related factors that contributed to the spread of EVD in Monrovia. The study was unique because I explored what it takes to cope with the threat of EVD and how government decrees such as mandatory cremation and regulation such as the banning of a public gathering of Monrovians may have influenced the spread of EVD. The findings generated new understanding of EVD survivors' and family caregivers' experiences of caring for sick relatives and being affected by EVD. Results may provide insight into better epidemic response during future EVD outbreaks.

I also explored the experiences of EVD survivors and family caregivers and provided a basis for better preparation of health care workers during future outbreaks. The findings may contribute towards more comprehensive health care policy changes and protocols that can better address the health needs of the affected patients, the survivors, and the general public. This research study may contribute to positive social and policy change by providing an enhanced understanding of what it is to be affected by EVD. It explained the experiences of survivors and family caregivers, including officials of government, NGO staff, academicians, and reporters from the media which broadened the public's understanding of what it means to be affected by EVD. This new knowledge may change people's overall perceptions and beliefs about EVD.

Since the initial outbreaks of EVD in the Democratic Republic of Congo (DRC) and Sudan in 1976, healthcare practitioners have been challenged to contain EVD, thus posing a global threat of spreading the EVD (Bellizzi, 2014; Gomes et al., 2014). This study makes an original contribution by improving on the knowledge gap in the literature geared to creating an efficient mechanism to contain EVD, which will add to the existing knowledge that key policy-makers and health practitioners rely upon to make decisions. It is also anticipated that this study may contribute to positive social change by providing insight into improved policies and training practices for healthcare practitioners on appropriate intervention techniques to effectively contain EVD.

SUMMARY

I examined the social, economic, and policy factors that contributed to the spread of the 2014 EVD outbreak in the city of Monrovia. I used a case study approach that falls within the qualitative case study research tradition. I conducted in-depth interviews, observations, and documentation of participants in three communities that were the hardest hit by the 2014 EVD outbreak in Monrovia. I designed this study to understand how EVD survivors, family caregivers and the general public coped with the threat of the 2014 EVD outbreak. I explored the understanding of the general public as it relates to the reality of EVD. Chapter 1 introduced the study and explained the background of the study. It also outlined the main issues related to EVD including social, economic, and policy factors that contributed to the spread of EVD. The research design and method including the theoretical framework guiding the study was also highlighted.

In Chapter 2, I focus on the review of the literature that supports the study. Also in Chapter 2, I highlighted the guiding theoretical framework for the study and presented an overview of EVD. The data collection process was discussed including the CDC classification of EVD. The literature in Chapter 2 relates to several factors for spreading EVD, these factors are highlighted and fully discussed. Chapter 2 was then concluded by discussing the gap in the study and the current healthcare and policy initiatives health care practitioners adopted to contain EVD.

CHAPTER 2

REVIEW OF LITERATURE

INTRODUCTION

The purpose of this qualitative case study was to explore the social-cultural, economic, poverty, and policy factors that contributed to the spread of the 2014 EVD outbreak in Liberia (WHO, 2015). In this regard, it is critical to first develop a clear perception about the concepts related to EVD. The literature reviewed for this study were synthesized from the most current and relevant information on EVD.

The following are the 12 main themes that formed the basis for this study: (a) overview of EVD, (b) the theoretical framework guiding the study, (c) strategies used to collect data, (d) the Centers for Disease Control and Prevention (CDC) classification of EVD, (e) poverty and cultural factors that led to the transmission and spread of EVD, (f) seasonal outbreaks of EVD, (g) case management and prevention practices, (h) the role of media during epidemics, (i) the role of governments and community reactions, (j) fear and denial of EVD, (k) gaps in the study, and (l) current healthcare and policy initiatives. The literature reviewed in this chapter was an attempt to collect and organize what is already known about EVD. The literature largely focused on the social-cultural, economic, poverty, and policy factors for spreading EVD, including life experience accounts of survivors and family caregivers who coped with the threat of EVD under highly stigmatized conditions. The literature then highlighted coping strategies, clinical care interventions, and needs of affected individuals.

OVERVIEW OF EBOLA VIRUS DISEASE

According to (World Health Organization [WHO], 2014), the first 2 EVD outbreaks simultaneously occurred in 1976 in Nzara, Sudan, and Yambuku, Democratic Republic of Congo (DRC). The Sudan outbreak occurred in a village near the Ebola River from which the disease got its name. The Sudan EVD outbreak infected over 284 people and recorded a mortality rate of 53%. The DRC outbreak infected over 318 people and recorded the highest mortality rate of 88% (Jones, 2011). The CDC (2014) confirmed and WHO (2014) concurred that EVD comprises five species including the; (a) Bundibugyo Ebolavirus (BEBOV), (b) Zaire Ebolavirus (ZEBOV), (c) Sudan Ebolavirus (SEBOV), (d) Reston Ebolavirus (REBOV), and (e) Tai Forest Virus (TAFV, formerly, Cote d'Ivoire Ebolavirus). The above EVD subtypes were named after the country or location in which the virus was first identified or isolated (Jones, 2011; WHO, 2014).

The 2014 EVD outbreaks in West Africa was the largest EVD outbreak in history. The outbreak started in Guinea and later spread into Sierra Leone and then into Liberia. Liberia, specifically the city of Monrovia, was the hardest hit by EVD recording over 4,808 deaths and 10,666 infections. According to WHO (2014), the first EVD case in Liberia was recorded on March 30, 2014, in the Foya district of Lofa County, Northern Liberia. According to LISGIS (2014), towns and villages in the Foya district are less populated as compared to the city of Monrovia which has a population of over 1 million people.

Past EVD outbreaks in other parts of Africa occurred in rural areas, and were controlled and stopped while they were still in the rural areas; where population density was lower, community ties were stronger, and measures to prevent transmission were easier to implement (Bellizzi, 2014). WHO (2015) argued that early recognition of EVD symptoms and isolation of the infected patients are the best ways to contain the spread of EVD. Bellizzi (2014) concurred with WHO (2014) and recounted the situation in Nigeria when a Liberian passenger infected with EVD flew to Nigeria on July 20, 2014, and was quickly detected and isolated. By then doctors and nurses in Nigeria who rushed to treat the affected patient from Liberia without PPE got infected as well. Subsequently, intense contact tracing attempts were made which led to the detection and isolation of infected secondary cases. These new cases were contained as well to bring to an immediate end the spread of EVD in Nigeria in the shortest possible time (Bellizzi 2014). Besides Guinea, Liberia, Nigeria, and Sierra Leone; Senegal was the fifth West African country to be affected with EVD. Senegal applied the same method as Nigeria did, and managed to rapidly contain EVD from spreading. A well-coordinated interagency effort can prove to be effective in the containment of EVD (Bellizzi, 2014).

DATA COLLECTION STRATEGIES

I conducted this literature review using mostly online databases such as EBSCO, ProQuest, SAGE, CINAHL Plus, PsycARTICLES, MEDLINE, ProQuest Nursing and Allied Health, and ProQuest Dissertations and Theses. I accessed these databases through the Walden University Library. I also used Ovid and PubMed to review e-books, journal articles in nursing, public health, medicine, and infectious diseases. Literature was reviewed from several journals, research articles, print books, as well as newsletters and newspapers.

These data have been carefully analyzed for relevance and meaningfulness, summarized and then categorized to focus the study. Therefore, by studying what has already been learned about EVD and the experiences of survivors and caregivers, I was able to identify a gap in the previous studies that raised the need for future research. Such study will contribute to positive social change through providing insight to support future of effective policies and intervention techniques to contain EVD during forthcoming outbreaks.

THEORETICAL FRAMEWORK

The guiding theoretical framework for this study was Bandura's social cognitive theory (SCT). Researchers using this theory believe that an individual can learn new knowledge by directly observing others within the context of social interactions, experiences, and media influences (Ertmer & Ottenbreit-Leftwich, 2010). SCT has provided evidence that comprehensive disease education is essential for containing an epidemic. This theory explained human behavior regarding the continuous reciprocal interaction between cognitive, behavioral, and environmental influences. The literature reviewed prevention-based disease education studies that have used the SCT to frame a change in the participants' behavior either to increase awareness or to recommend control mechanism (Roach et al., 2003). SCT emphasizes how cognitive, behavioral, personal, and environmental factors interact to determine motivation and behavior. To change the behavior, Bandura (1997) explained that an individual must first understand the social context that has shaped his or her behavior and then reverse their learning process.

The SCT was developed by Miller and Dollard in 1941 for the purpose of social learning. The SCT was later broadened in 1963 by Bandura and Walters with the principles of observational learning and vicarious reinforcement. The SCT was relevant for this study because it supported the research to explain how survivors and family caregivers coped with the threat of EVD during the 2014 outbreak in Liberia. The SCT examined the perception, emotional, and behavioral aspects for understanding behavioral change caused by the stigma EVD impacted on survivors and the general public (Bandura, 1997). This theory enables the researcher to fill in the gaps of how people coped with the threat of EVD. The SCT also allowed for other theoretical areas such as psychology to provide new insights and understanding of EVD. Dee Roo et al. (1995) used the social representation theory (SRT) to explore the behavior of EVD survivors in Kibale, Uganda, upon initially hearing that they have survived from EVD and declared Ebola-free.

Due to the constant challenges of coping with the threat and physical symptoms of EVD, survivors graced the news with distrust. The label "survivor" has stigmatized them and the news was received with cautiousness and hesitation. Helman (2007) explained that in situations such as EVD outbreaks, people respond differently, some will turn to their natural environment, and others will turn to supernatural forces for cure or healing. Helman (2007) noted that because of the great importance culture plays in ones live; it is crucial to understand the socio-cultural dimensions underlying people's health values, beliefs, and behaviors. The SCT subscribed to Helman's argument affirming that environment influenced the individual, and the individual influences the environment.

Furthermore, Miller and Morris (2014) outlined three basic concepts in the SCT: (a) that people can learn through observation and emulate those observed behaviors, (b) inner psychological states are a critical part of the education process, (c) and an individual skill acquisition does not necessarily equate to a change in behavior. Human self-regulatory capability plays the central role in SCT, as it does in other prominent theories of self-regulation and motivation (Stajkovic & Luthans, 1998b). Deci and Ryan (2002) argued that self-regulation is the highest level of learning which allows individuals to adjust their learning strategies to contextual and personal changes. In this regard, individuals may be able to start using strategies to adapt themselves to contextual and circumstantial characteristics and be motivated by self-efficacy perceptions of potential situations. In this direction, Bandura (1997) stated that self-efficacy belief serves as an important motivational source driven by an individual's judgment about his/her abilities to organize and perform some actions to achieve desirable goals and functions. Coping under the threat of EVD relates to the above argument as EVD survivors may have been stigmatized as a result of EVD.

According to SCT, people may set higher standards for themselves and activate future behaviors to satisfy the new standards (Bandura, 1997). The self-reflective capability in SCT can be defined as human self-reflective consciousness. Self-reflective consciousness enables people to think and analyze their experiences and thought processes. By reflecting on their different personal experiences, participants, health caregivers, and policy makers can generate knowledge about their environment and themselves.

Traditionally, one of the constructs most commonly equated with self-efficacy is self-esteem. Both are conceptually similar, but self-esteem and self-efficacy are different. The first difference is the domain that self-esteem and self-efficacy cover. Self-esteem is theoretically portrayed as a global construct that represents a person's self-evaluations across a wide variety of different situations. On the other hand, self-efficacy is the individual's belief about a task and-context-specific capability. Second, self-esteem tends to be more stable, almost trait like, whereas self-efficacy is state like, a dynamic construct which changes over time as new information and experiences are obtained. Self-esteem is based on an introspective, reflective evaluation of self. For example feelings of self-worth, that is usually derived from perceptions about several personal characteristics such as intelligence or integrity.

The literature reviewed indicated that most studies have largely focused on the social-cultural, economic, and policy factors for spreading EVD. There is a little or no literature that explains what it takes to cope with the threat of EVD. Questions such as how did government mandatory cremation policy and banning of public gatherings impact the spread of EVD, are yet to be answered. Using Yin's (2014) case study design, the SCT allowed the researcher to explore the answers to the above questions and how people acquire EVD, which may have resulted to stigma and behavioral changes of EVD survivors. This theory helped identify and explained intervention strategies in the context of Bandura (1997). The SCT ensures the evaluation of behavioral change during epidemics based on the social-cultural and beliefs of people. In general, the SCT provided a framework for designing, implementing, and evaluating the research. The SCT is primarily based on behavioral, personal, and environmental factors which were used to conduct this study.

FACTORS FOR TRANSMISSION AND SPREAD OF EBOLA VIRUS DISEASE

The review of the literature for this study explored many social-cultural, economic, and the traditional aspects of how EVD has been spread in Africa. I explored the challenges both the communities and health care providers faced in understanding and containing the disease (WHO, 2015). I also clarified from the literature review that poverty helped to influence the past and the 2014 EVD outbreaks in West Africa (Jones, 2011). The literature review further explained other types of research that focused on the impact of EVD in Africa based on the main themes for this study. Since the initial outbreaks of EVD in 1976 in Sudan and the DRC and to the recent 2014 EVD outbreaks in West Africa, the concept of culture has always played a significant role in the spread of EVD (WHO, 2015).

Hewlett and Amola (2003) defined culture as an integrated pattern of learned beliefs and behaviors people share as a tradition or their way of life. These may include their way of thinking, their styles of communication, ways of interaction, views, and roles of relationships, values, practices and customs. In a traditional setting, culture set aside rules and scripts of how certain people should live in society. Culture helps people make decisions during the course of their lives by applying rules handed down from generation to generation. Helman (2007) affirmed that due to the complex nature of human relationships and especially how people are intricately influenced by their backgrounds, a person's culture is often the inherited habit in which he or she perceives and understands the world. According to Helman (2007), in situations such as EVD outbreaks, people respond differently, some will turn to their natural environment, and others will turn to supernatural forces for cure or healing. Helman (2007) noted that because of the great importance culture plays in ones live, it is crucial to understanding the socio-cultural dimensions underlying people's health values, beliefs, and behaviors. Helman (2007) stressed that this practice will ensure successful patient clinical outcomes during disease outbreaks such as EVD.

WHO (2014) provided evidence that cultural beliefs and practices affected patients' attitudes about medical care whenever an outbreak occurred. Local dwellers specifically people who live in remote towns and villages rely on their culture to guide their livelihood. These local dwellers lack the ability to understand, manage and cope with the course of a strange illness, the meaning of a diagnosis, and the consequences of medical treatment (Helman, 2007). In agreement with Helman (2007), WHO (2014) much like Hewlett and Amola (2003) affirmed that cultural beliefs and practices significantly influence individuals' perceptions of health and illnesses. Culture poses challenges for recognition of symptoms, an impact of illness, communication of symptoms to caregivers including their understanding of the management strategies, expectations of care and adherence to preventive measures and medications (WHO, 2014). Culturally generated values influenced individuals and families roles and expectations during past EVD outbreaks (Helman, 2007). These cultural values or beliefs dictated how they used information about EVD and treatment, and how they manage their dead loved ones (Helman, 2007). Cultural beliefs and practices impede western preventive efforts and delay or complicate medical care. This can result to health care workers using remedies that can be either beneficial or harmful to affected individuals (Hewlett and Amola, 2003).

The positive or negative effects of the beliefs arise from the wide range of understandings people have around what causes a particular disease. In communities worldwide, various explanatory models are used to understand disease causation. These models and the accompanying belief systems vary widely, from witchcraft to virus and weak immunity (Hewlett and Amola, 2003). Western ideology perceives the human body to be an intricate machine which should be maintained at all times to ensure effectiveness. Illness, on the other hand, is perceived as anti to the good functioning of the body. However, from a traditional point of view, this western ideology contrasts widely with African ideology about illness and cause of illness and death (Helman, 2007).

In Liberia, like most parts of Sub-Saharan Africa, cultural groups have built explanatory frameworks to defend the etiology of different diseases. Hewlett and Amola (2003) argued that most Africans believe in spirits as their guiding forces. These spirits which are believed to be either 'good' or 'bad' impact human lives in both good and bad ways. That is, the good spirits are believed to protect humans against harm, misfortune or disease; whereas the bad spirits would inflict disease, misfortune or suffering (Hewlett and Amola, 2003).

This belief system is structured around the notion that protection from the spirits is directed at individuals who respect social, cultural and religious rituals and practices. They believe that when individuals or families who abandon the norms of the good spirits risk being turned over to the bad spirits for punishment (Hewlett and Amola, 2003). Helman (2007) confirmed that these models hold that disease may result from an internal imbalance within the body or may arise from negative external influences related to actions of bad spirits, witches or deities.

Foster (1976) expounded that the cause of disease outbreaks in Sub-Saharan Africa can be explained in two categories: naturalistic category and personality category. The naturalistic category relates to the natural causes of illness. According to Foster (1976), the naturalistic category explains simple illnesses such as headaches, muscle aches, and fevers whose cause is almost always specific. In this case, the sick person or a close family member is expected to seek help from a traditional healer who is skilled and knowledgeable in symptomatic treatment. The traditional healer is also knowledgeable in local remedies such as herbs, food restrictions, and massages, among others, to correct such imbalance or illness. In contrast, the personalistic category relates to others, including the supernatural actors. In this category as Foster (1976) explained disease causation occurs as a result of active, purposeful intervention of an agent who is believed to be a supernatural being such as; a deity or god, a ghost or evil spirit, a witch or sorcerer (Foster, 1976).

The sick person is seen primarily as a victim, the object of aggression or punishment directed specifically against them for reasons that concern them alone. Hewlett and Amola (2003) agreed with Foster (1976) and added that most cultures in Sub-Saharan Africa, believe that individuals become prone to illness if they do not conform to certain personal or social standards or if they misbehave or breach taboos, customs, and traditions expected of them or their parents. The implication is that people who become afflicted by a strange but serious disease may be exposed to punishment by the spirits or gods. Such affliction is self-made and may be a worthy punishment for failure to abide by norms, thereby leading to their ostracism and neglect (Hewlett and Amola, 2003).

Foster (1976) concurred with Hewlett and Amola (2003) that the affected person or close relatives are expected to seek traditional healers with supernatural powers and skills. The primary concern of the patient and their family is not the immediate cause of illness, but rather who is responsible for their illness, and why did it happen to them (Foster, 1976). At this point, the diagnostic process starts with the traditional healer who is believed to have supernatural powers. The healer is perceived to have direct contact with the spirit world, from which he or she invokes magical powers to find out who was responsible for the disease and why the victim was afflicted (Foster, 1976).

After the 'who' and 'why' have been determined, Foster (1976) explained that the treatment for the immediate cause may be administered by the same person (healer), or the task may be referred to a lesser healer, often a known herbalist which may require offering some gifts to their ancestors or gods. The traditional healer will then recommend that the patient or family members perform a ritual in order to remove the 'who' or 'why' by sacrificing a white chicken, sheep or goat for the purpose of pleasing their ancestors or gods and chase away the offending evil spirits (Foster, 1976).

Hewlett and Amola (2003) recounted the interactions of some local people (villagers) and international healthcare workers as it relate to blood drawn for laboratory testing. The villagers raised concern about how these international healthcare workers would come to their villages to collect blood from them and their children but never return to give results. The villagers also complained that some of their children would die after the collection of their blood. The locals believed that the blood was harvested for sale in Switzerland (Hewlett and Amola, 2003).

According to Hewlett and Amola (2003), traditional healers claimed they can heal any disease including EVD. They (traditional healers) use their visionary power to see and encounter the disease. Hewlett and Amola (2003) noted that not all traditional healers can heal EVD and other related diseases because they have to encounter the spirits and the spirits are too strong to face. Therefore, only special and very powerful healers are favored by the spirits (gods) and can communicate with them and bring healings (Hewlett and Amola, 2003).

Although there might be traditional or cultural factors that influenced the spread of EVD, poverty also played a significant role in the spread of the virus in West Africa (Chan, 2014). For over a decade, Guinea, Liberia, and Sierra Leone have been challenged to maintain political stability. Liberia, in particular, has just returned to political stability in 2006 after a 14-year civil war that destroyed its infrastructure including hospitals and schools (WHO, 2014). As affirmed by Chan (2014), the destruction or lack of standard health facilities and trained medical staff in Liberia made it difficult to contain the 2014 EVD outbreak. Containment measures such as early detection and isolations of cases, contact tracing, and monitoring, and meticulous procedures for infection control were impeded (Chan, 2014). In addition, WHO (2014) affirmed that there is currently no vaccine and no defined curative treatment for EVD. In this vein, Chan (2014) agreed that the implementation of the above containment measures has successfully brought previous EVD outbreaks under control. However, WHO (2014) also noted that with these control measures in place and working effectively, EVD still remain a difficult disease to diagnose, since early symptoms of EVD mimic those of several commonly known diseases such as; malaria, lassa fever, and typhoid fever in West Africa. WHO (2014) explained that by the time the patients' condition is accurately diagnosed, EVD has incubated, thus making it very difficult to treat.

Despite these cultural beliefs and sporadic cultural challenges that policy makers and healthcare practitioners encounter when responding to an epidemic such as EVD, the primary concern for scientists, healthcare workers and policy makers remain to find a defined control mechanism and cure for

EVD. It is against this background that Bellizzi (2014) described the three main interventions techniques such as (a) coordination, (b) isolation and treatment, and (c) contact tracings and follow-ups. These techniques were effectively used to contain past EVD outbreaks in 1976 when the virus first appeared in Sudan and the DRC (Bellizzi, 2014). Bellizzi stressed the need for coordination between isolation and treatment during an EVD outbreak. In this regard, responding to EVD cases involves a correct coordination between isolation and treatment, contact tracing and follow-up of each contact for 21 days after exposure (Bellizzi, 2014). Bellizzi (2014) further argued that the process should also involve the strategic use of laboratories in order to reduce the chances of hospital amplification of EVD in resource-limited health systems such as in Liberia, particularly the city of Monrovia.

According to Chan (2014), most Liberians do not have steady or salaried jobs, thus leaving them to involve into petty trades. Liberians, in general, depend on Monrovia (Monrovia is the capital city of Liberia) for trade and jobs, thus causing a fluid population movement across the country which may have exposed the city to the high rate of EVD infections and mortality during the 2014 EVD outbreak. Like Guinea and Sierra Leone, Liberia is among the poorest countries in the world. WHO (2014) quoting the World Bank Human Development Index (HDI) stated that over 85% of Liberians live on less than one dollar per day and cannot afford to buy the cheapest over-the-counter medication. According to WHO (2014), life expectancy for male in Liberia is 56 years, and for a female is 59 years (2014 estimate). Chan (2014) noted that with such vulnerability, Liberians remain ill-equipped to fight a disease like EVD.

Coupled with all the above challenges, Liberia has just emerged from a 14-year civil war that destroyed most of its infrastructure including hospitals, clinics, and schools; thus leaving a generation of children without education, and access to better medical facilities. In most counties of Liberia, only one or two doctors are available for every 100,000 people (Chan, 2014). Isolation wards and even hospital capacity for infection control are virtually non-existent in these affected countries. Contacts of infected persons are being traced but not consistently isolated for monitoring (Chan, 2014). Chowell and Nishiura (2014) provided a supporting side to the argument, and stated that the lack of public health infrastructures, timely resources, and control measures, including the absence of epidemiological surveillance for the timely identification of case clusters at health care centers in Guinea, Liberia, and Sierra Leone helped the spread of the 2014 EVD in West Africa.

According to Chowell and Nishiura (2014), EVD is introduced into the human population through close contact with the blood, secretions, organs or other bodily fluids of infected animals such as chimpanzees, gorillas, fruit bats, monkeys, forest antelope, and porcupines found ill or dead in the rainforest. EVD then spread through human-to-human transmission by direct contact (via broken skin or mucous membranes) with the blood, secretions, organs or other bodily fluids of infected people. In homes or hospital settings, the virus is further spread through the fluids of infected people via contaminated beddings and clothing. Healthcare workers were infected while treating patients with suspected or confirmed EVD (Chowell & Nishiura, 2014).

EVD infection occurred through close contact with patients when infection control precautions were not strictly practiced. Infected individuals remain infectious as long as their blood contains the virus (WHO, 2014). Once an individual is infected with EVD, the incubation period ranges from 2 to 21 days. The infected person becomes contagious after developing symptoms of EVD, and those that have earlier provided care without the use of personal protective equipment (PPE) stand the risk of being infected as well. Usually, larger outbreaks have tended to occur after infected individuals enter low quality health care systems where health care workers lack the capacity and necessary PPE to control and contain EVD (Jones, 2011).

According to Tosh and Sampathkumar (2014), it is critical to understand the unending risks of transmission dynamics and resurgence of EVD. Ensuring this understanding will help in implementing rapid and effective response interventions designed to specific local settings and context. Community understanding of the clinical presentation, clinical course, transmission, and prevention of EVD can help reduce anxiety, panic, and stigma associated with the disease and allow healthcare providers to confidently provide medical care to individuals suspected of having EVD (Tosh & Sampathkumar, 2014).

Much like Tosh and Sampathkumar (2014), Tambo (2014) found that the 1976 EVD outbreak was a result of humans who made contact with infected animals. Subsequently, most of the 2014 EVD outbreaks in West Africa occurred because of direct contact with infected family members. Family caregivers or healthcare providers were exposed to the mucous membranes or broken skin with blood or body fluids of an infected relative or patient. When a person is infected with EVD, blood, sweat, feces, and vomit becomes highly infectious. Health care workers and family caregivers who come in close contact with infected individuals with EVD without proper use of PPE are at highest risk for secondary infection.

Farmer (2001) interjected that the spread of the 1976 EVD in the DRC and Sudan was also caused by substandard medical practices in hospitals. Seemingly health workers at the time were using dirty needles (used needles) on patients. Farmer (2001) further explained that five needles were used on 300-600 patients per day, thus transmitting EVD into other patients who may not have actually contracted EVD from the beginning. The spread of EVD in past and recent outbreaks was also influenced by regional trade networks and other evolving social systems (WHO, 2014). Farmer (2001) stressed that all EVD outbreaks have proven to mostly affect those living in poverty. WHO (2014) concurred with Farmer (2001) and added that like most infectious diseases, EVD-affected countries or regions have low quality health care systems, where health care providers served poor people and family members are the sole attendants to their sick relatives.

Famer (2001) further argued that despite these detrimental medical, cultural, and social or traditional practices that may have influenced the transmission and spread of EVD, extreme poverty cannot be ruled out. The affected countries are known for their dysfunctional healthcare systems, coupled with mistrust of government officials after years of armed conflicts. Impoverished communities are vulnerable to disease outbreaks due to unsanitary conditions. Unattended water ponds in communities serve as breeding grounds for many disease infestations such as malaria, and typhoid fever (Farmer, 2001).

WHO (2015) added that under these grave conditions, EVD infection into humans is common during outbreaks since residents of these areas live and transact daily businesses around these potential disease reservoirs. Farmer (2001) stressed that preventing future epidemic outbreaks in poor resource countries such as Guinea, Liberia, and Sierra Leone should first begin by creating a healthy community. Continuous disease education should be prioritized on a daily basis before an outbreak occurs. This should include daily radio education of preventable disease strategies. Posters, banners, flyers, and brochures bearing disease prevention messages in order to prepare the communities in cases of an outbreak should be distributed to the general public (Farmer, 2001). WHO (2015) agreed with Farmer (2001) and added that disease education should also include best burial practices whenever an epidemic occurs. As noted by the CDC (2014), Feldmann and Geisbert (2012), Leroy et al. (2005) and WHO (2014), the actual origin or reservoir for EVD remain unknown, but most studies point to human-to-animal contact as the source of EVD. The disease than is introduced into human settings and transmitted from one infected person to another and to a large scale of infections.

According to Tosh and Sampathkumar (2014), most rural residents depend on the forest for food thus exposing them to eating of bush meat which is scientifically proven to be the reservoir for EVD. These village dwellers also depend on animal skins for costumes and other activities such as sacrifices to their gods. Tosh and Sampathkumar (2014) significantly noted that in Liberia and West Africa as a whole, about almost the entire population living in bigger towns and cities eat some sort of bushmeat and other forest grown fruits. Most residents in cities would buy arts and crafts made from animal parts including the skins for in home interior decoration. All these activities as Tosh and Sampathkumar (2014) explained exposed humans to potential EVD contamination.

The main issues of concern here according to Tosh and Sampathkumar (2014) are the questions of how to contain, cure, and prevent the spread of EVD when it does occur; taking into consideration that all EVD outbreaks have occurred in poor regions of Africa. In this context, Tosh and Sampathkumar (2014) explained that there are several challenges in delivering best care that are well upstream of treatment centers established to handle EVD outbreaks. Several studies indicate and Tosh and Sampathkumar (2014) agreed that social mobilization and community health education during epidemics of high mortality is challenged by community mistrust. The first thing to do in this situation as argued by Tosh and Sampathkumar (2014) is trying to get the communities to accept the illness and the necessities for clinical care. In all cases, the impact of an effective social mobilization and community health education efforts are impeded by poor health care systems, such as in Guinea, Liberia, and Sierra Leone.

As stated by Chan (2014) and affirmed by Gomes et al. (2014), population mobility which involved the movement of people trading or looking for jobs or looking for safer areas from EVD, better health infrastructure, or food seriously influenced the disease propagation and plays a major role in spreading EVD and in the effectiveness of any intervention strategy. It is critical to understand these patterns of movements when planning interventions strategies designed to contain EVD and further outbreaks (Gomes et al., 2014). While the primary goal of any outbreak is to stop it as quickly as possible, it is difficult to accomplish such goal when individuals are traveling from EVD-affected town or village to another (Gomes et al., 2014).

CASE MANAGEMENT AND PREVENTION PRACTICES

Managing and containing EVD remains a daunting challenge, partially due to the fact that the natural reservoir of the virus remains unknown, thus making it difficult to institute primary prevention measures (Jones, 2011). Leroy et al. (2005) suggested that in the absence of an effective primary prevention technique, the main epidemic management should rely on educating the communities about EVD. During EVD outbreaks, traditional practices such as burial rites should be suspended and enforced in agreement with those who practice these rites. Hygiene practices such as washing of hands and avoiding handshakes should be reinforced as means to contain the spread of EVD (Jones, 2011).

According to WHO (2015), the spread of EVD in many cases correlates with African culture and belief systems. Many Africans reject biomedicine, resorting to traditional healers and sorcerers whom they believed can cure their illness. The use of traditional medicine is rooted in African history, even before the outbreaks of EVD. Due to poor access to public health centers, care by traditional healers or self-medication through pharmacies (over-the-counter drugs) have become the most preferred option for many poor West Africans. Most West Africans believed that hospitals are places of contagion and death further reinforcing their need for traditional medicine (WHO, 2015). Many health centers are constructed with high fences and sometimes draped barbed wire, which many community members perceived as a prison center instead of a place for health care and healing (Hodge et al., 2014).

Performing traditional burial rites is another source of transmitting EVD. WHO (2015) stressed that these practices should be suspended during EVD outbreaks. Jones (2011) and WHO (2015) examined those behavioral practices such as traditional medicine, funeral rites, culture, beliefs, and hunting and eating of bushmeat that may have attributed to the spread of the 2014 EVD outbreaks in West Africa. Like previous EVD outbreaks which occurred in equatorial Africa, the 2014 West African EVD outbreaks were characterized by high-risk behaviors. Most residents of these affected countries believed in ancestral funeral and burial rites. Medical anthropologists noted that these practices fueled large explosions of new cases on a daily basis; as health care providers struggled to contain the spread of EVD outbreaks.

According to WHO (2014), the Guinea Ministry of Health reported that about 60% of EVD cases were linked to traditional burial and funeral practices. The same or higher percentages were also respectively reported by the Liberia and Sierra Leone health authorities. WHO also confirmed that their staff in Sierra Leone estimated that over 80% of cases were caused by traditional practices (WHO, 2014). Traditional burial practices in Guinea, Liberia and Sierra Leone are reinforced by several secret societies, where some mourners are required to bathe in or anoint others with water from the washing of their deceased. Some mourners are required by norms to sleep by their dead relative for several nights believing that doing so allows the transfer of powers (WHO, 2014). A deep-seated cultural trait in West Africa is compassion. Most West African cultures stressed the need for compassion for their ill relatives and ceremonial care for their bodies if they die (Jones, 2011).

WHO (2014) interjected that individuals from the 2014 EVD-affected countries rely on farming for their livelihood. This may have exposed them to contact with animals. Cross-border trade is a significant way of life in this region. WHO (2015) reported that population mobility in these countries is seven times higher than anywhere in the world. Poverty is the driving force behind the grave population movement as people travel daily across porous borders trading goods and looking for work or food. Many extended West African families also have relatives living in their neighboring countries (Hodge et al., 2014). To respond to EVD outbreak, certain requirements must be met and this process could incur certain challenges. WHO (2015) agreed with Hodge et al. (2014) and recommended that EVD-affected countries should evaluate and intensify their respective national public health emergency preparedness and response plans and national command and coordination structures. To accomplish this, countries should adapt an incident management structure (IMS) and emergency operations center (EOC) to reinforce emergency health operations. This should include validating their respective national emergency response plan for emerging infectious diseases through simulation exercises. Case management is critical in this direction (WHO, 2015).

WHO (2015) further stressed the need for health workers to recognize their obligations at all times to provide best medical care to improve patient survival. This will ensure symptom relief and palliation when need be. Especially during epidemics such as EVD, clinical care must be strengthened while reducing the risk of transmitting the disease to others, including health care workers. In this regard, it is crucial for health care workers to comprehend EVD and adhere to best practices of infection control during outbreaks and even after (WHO, 2015). According to WHO (2015), it is important to avoid the unprotected handling of dead bodies infected with EVD. Doing this will constitute a biosafety hazard.

THE ROLE OF GOVERNMENT AND COMMUNITY REACTIONS TO EBOLA VIRUS DISEASE

Community resistance also influenced the spread of the 2014 EVD. The misperception about the mysterious disease caused many to believe that EVD is not real. Many residents of Liberia in particular, believe that EVD is not real (Chan, 2014). WHO (2015) noted that these individuals argued that they and their ancestors have been living in the same ecological environment for centuries, hunting and eating the same animals and never got infected with EVD. Chan (2014) and WHO (2015) recounted some of the measures community members in Monrovia instituted to control human movements and to prevent the spread of EVD.

According to Chan (2014), community members became afraid to allow and host anybody from another community or neighbor into their homes, even if the visitor was their own relative. Communities were apprehensive of the

Liberian government to handle their affairs as it relates to EVD (Chan, 2014). Communities' resistance grew stronger when their loved ones were buried or cremated without their consent or participation of ancestral mourning rites, resulting to public outcry and demonstration.

Another reason for the spread of EVD in Liberia was due to strikes by hospital staff and burial teams. These strikes were due to the failure of the government of Liberia to pay healthcare workers for several weeks or months. Some of the strikes were also because of lack of PPE which resulted to deaths of health workers. Dead bodies were left in the streets for several days, thus further escalating the spread of EVD. From all indications, EVD remains a global challenge with no definite answer to containing EVD when an outbreak does occur. This is particularly important given West Africa's vulnerability to future outbreaks (WHO 2015).

Community resistance and noncompliance with governments, local, and international health workers was mainly due to the lack of knowledge about the cause of EVD. Their lack of knowledge caused them to deny the existence of EVD and linked the cause of the epidemic to witchcraft or a government conspiracy theory. According to Chowell and Nishiura (2014), most Liberians believed that the 2014 EVD outbreak was created by their government to gain control of population or to solicit monetary assistance from the international community. These ideologies made some residents of Monrovia to loot and destroy quarantining centers. The looters took away their sick relatives and hid them from the government, which further exacerbated the spread of EVD (Chowell & Nishiura, 2014).

WHO (2014) explained that the Liberian government reacted to the spreading of EVD by banning public gatherings including the closure of schools, businesses and places of worship. According to WHO (2014), several local Liberian newspapers published horrific headlines such as this one by the Inquirer entitled, "Liberia police fire on protesters as West Africa's Ebola toll hits 1, 350" (Inquirer, 2014, p. 1). This report was referencing the Liberian government's decree that quarantined the entire West Point community. Residents of the West Point community challenged the government's decree and decided to go out in such of food, which led to the police shooting. The Liberian government also announced a nationwide curfew as means to contain the spread of EVD (WHO, 2014).

Community resistance in this situation was based on government ineptitude and mistrust. West African governments, in general, are corrupt and unreliable which provoked the public outcry. These governments have led their people for over a century and have never been willing to establish a standard hospital or clinic despite all the international assistance. Instead, governments from these affected countries used the armed forces to enforce epidemic control measures and to quarantine communities, which further provoked public resentment. Communities were quarantined without government assistance of food, water, and other necessities to support women and children (Chan, 2014).

WHO (2015) added that the burial process is a sensitive issue for family members and the community as a whole, which in most cases draw resistance and conflict. Therefore, it is important to initially have the family informed about the procedure and ensure they fully understand. This may help to avoid the hard feelings associated with traditional burial rites, religious, and personal rights. These steps can play a pivotal role in the containment and prevention of EVD when carefully and strictly enforced (WHO, 2015).

FEAR AND DENIAL OF EBOLA VIRUS DISEASE

Denial and fears are the main feelings for EVD survivors, and believing in God was the source of hope for survivals (De Roo et al., 1995). Fear during an epidemic is one of the most difficult barriers to overcome. WHO (2014) affirmed that fear causes infected individuals to escape from surveillance facilities. According to De Roo et al. (1995), fear gripped communities when they began to see government employees setting up fever check-points and disinfecting their homes which they (residents) believed resulted into them getting sick. Fear further gripped the communities when they saw people dressed in something that looked like spacesuits who took their sick relatives to hospitals or into barricaded tent-like structures from which many never returned home. Family members tend to hide symptomatic relatives or take them to traditional healers. De Roo et al. (1995) exerted that fear impacts patients, family members, and healthcare providers during epidemic such as EVD.

During the 2014 EVD outbreaks in West Africa, more than 170 health workers were infected and 81 of them died in the first six months of the outbreak, thus causing healthcare workers to fear for their lives. Because of EVD fear in 2014, airlines canceled their flights into EVD declared countries. This action by the airlines companies made it difficult for healthcare workers and medical supplies to be transported to these countries, thus further exacerbating the spread of EVD (WHO, 2014). Fear from a positive point of view leads to a very high level of vigilance and clinical suspicion worldwide (De Roo et al., 1995).

According to WHO (2014), EVD fear has caused several false alarms at airports or even in hospital emergency rooms, which gave rise to early detection and prompt attention to patients. De Roo et al. (1995) argued that because there is no defined containment mechanism and cure for EVD, fear has become the first defense for family members to care for their sick relatives. They would prefer taking their sick ones to traditional healers who is believed to have powers to heal. Some community members would rather keep their sick relatives at home and then look up to God for healing to come, instead of taking them to government run quarantining centers, which they believed is a prison for death (WHO, 2014).

De Roo et al. (1995) explained that epidemics such as EVD impact individuals with fear, altruism, and stigma. These three significant human experiences dictate community reactions in responding to treatment and containment procedures. De Roo et al. (1995) noted that whenever there is fear in a situation like disease outbreaks, it set in motion two parallel processes namely; epidemiological and social processes.

The epidemiological process involves investigations undertaking by authorities to find out what is responsible for the etiological agent, who is at risk of infection, through which activities, and what can be done to reduce such risk. Health authorities need this epidemiological information to draw a clear picture in order to design appropriate containment and control mechanism during disease outbreaks. The social process is the psychological effect EVD inflicts on its victims, healthcare providers, and the affected communities. De Roo et al. (1995) further recounted that the 1976 EVD outbreak in Sudan was characterized by fear, alarm and panic among hospital staff.

Fear gripped health workers in Sudan when 61 of 154 nurses fell ill from EVD of whom 33 died. Health workers were also victims in the 1995 EVD outbreak in Zaire. It is reported that 25% of the 315 EVD cases were nursing staff. The fear of infection caused many nurses and other health workers to quit their jobs. Those health workers who bravely stayed became stigmatized because community members detested them for fear of being carriers of EVD. In some cases, some of these health workers were chased out of their homes and stones were thrown at them (De Roo et al., 1995). Fear for this study can be defined as a feeling of apprehension or alarm in response to an external source of danger. In this vein, according to (De Roo et al., 1995) health workers who bravely stayed to challenge EVD despite its deadly impact were obviously altruistic people.

De Roo et al. (1995) interjected that the proximity of health care facilities and bad roads condition also significantly influenced the 2014 EVD outbreaks in West Africa and Liberia in particular. De Roo et al. (1995) added that health facilities are miles away from most towns and villages, and motor roads are bad or non-existent. Emergency medical transportation services and telecommunication systems are poor or non-existent. These poor conditions greatly delayed communication and transportation of patients to treatment centers and laboratories (Hodge et al., 2014). In most cases, patients were transported to hospitals or health centers by means of public transport such as a taxi or bus. These vehicles continue their normal routine by transporting other passengers without being disinfected, thus creating the corridor of infecting other passengers with EVD. In other cases, family members take several days to walk their sick relatives to hospital or clinic, thus exposing them to contracting EVD (Hodge et al., 2014).

For these and other reasons, most rural residents would first prefer seeking the help of a traditional or spiritual healer for their illness. Their confidence in first seeking traditional healers as argued by Chowell and Nishiura (2014) is propelled by the lack of trust in government and denial of the existence of EVD. Lamontagne et al. (2014) agreed that because there is currently no vaccine or effective drugs to cure EVD, available drugs are at the experimental stage. Therefore, there is no assurance that patients who receive the experimental drugs will survive thus prompting fear in communities. This was evidence during all EVD outbreaks when some patients died while others survive (WHO, 2014). Because of this development, local dwellers especially those in towns and villages chose to turn to their gods for cure and protection against EVD (De Roo et al., 1995). A retrospective of past EVD outbreaks, when communities (villages) considered themselves abandoned, their only hope for survival was to turn to their gods. During epidemics such as EVD when government relationship with communities is characterized with mistrust, coupled with the challenge of finding effective containment mechanism and cure; people turn to belief in the existence of an omnipotent God for whom nothing is impossible (Lamontagne et al., 2014).

It is against this background that Lamontagne et al. (2014) researched the beliefs in god or spirits versus clinical intervention and provided literature indicating that the lack of resources and supportive care for EVD patients led to the high incidence of mortality. The 2014 EVD outbreaks occurred in very poor countries such as Guinea, Liberia and Sierra Leone where over 85% of the population is illiterate. These countries lack standard medical facilities to combat epidemics such as EVD (Lamontagne et al., 2014). According to Lamontagne et al. (2014), the concept of virus or disease and illness, in West Africa in general, is frequently associated with the world of the spirits (gods). West Africans believe these gods or spirits are either good or bad, and they impact human lives in both good and bad ways. That is, the good gods or spirits are believed to protect humans against harm, misfortune or disease; whereas the bad gods or spirits would inflict disease, misfortune or suffering. This belief system is structured around the notion that protection from the gods or spirits is directed at individuals who respect social, cultural and religious rituals and practices. Those individuals who abandon the norms of the good gods or spirits risk being turned over to the bad gods or spirits for punishment (Hewlett & Amola, 2003).

As means to differentiate myths from facts about EVD, De Roo et al. (1995), suggested that EVD awareness and education designed to win the confidence and support of rural residents should first be put into effect while awaiting the invention of EVD vaccine and or cure. Since human-to-animal contact is the foundation for EVD, rural residents should be educated to these facts. According to WHO (2015), malaria is prevalence in this region of West Africa and poses challenges during EVD outbreaks. Fever and vomiting are early symptoms of both malaria and EVD. Before EVD, communities were aware of these malaria symptoms. Based on this, relatives of patients would first begin to treat their loved ones with malaria drugs. In Liberia, many clinics or hospitals lack the appropriate diagnostic equipment to differentiate malaria from EVD, and patients showing signs of fever and vomiting were treated with malaria drugs. This situation usually present for the late care of EVD patients. Until the arrival and installation of international standard laboratories, patients were left with no medical hope but to hope in god (Lamontagne et al., 2014).

WHO (2015) concurred with Lamontagne et al. (2014) and added that after the arrival and installation of standard laboratories in Liberia, the next major issue was the lack of beds. Most patients were turned away. Patients were laid on floors in hallways and other areas of the health centers. However, WHO (2015) stressed that despite the above conditions and the fact that there is no cure for EVD, a supportive clinical care such as oral rehydration and intravenous fluid was provided which helped some patients to survive. Lamontagne et al. (2014) argued that this support was most effective than believing in god since there is no record of any kind that indicates a traditional healer or pastor or man of god curing anyone of EVD. There is evidence that healthcare workers can be protected against EVD infection once they use the appropriate PPE and follow strict intervention procedures (Lamontagne et al., 2014). According to Lamontagne et al. (2014), it is critical to recall that although survivors of most serious illness are known to react differently, individuals with a strong sense of spirituality tend to cope better with the aftereffects of life-threatening illness, presenting with a lesser psychological burden than others. Accordingly, family caregivers should assess changes in their relatives' spiritual beliefs and practices to help identify the need for spiritual counseling and support especially for those survivors perceived to be in a spiritual crisis (Lamontagne et al., 2014).

CLASSIFICATION OF EBOLA VIRUS DISEASE

EVD has posed a deadly threat to mankind globally, and yet there is no cure or a defined control mechanism to contain the virus when an outbreak occurs (WHO, 2015). According to the CDC (2014), EVD has been classified as a Biosafety Risk Group 4 (BRG 4) agent. The BRG 4 is the CDC's highest scale of biosafety rating because it poses a high health risk to healthcare workers and the general public. Because of the ability of EVD to be transmitted naturally from animals to humans, Feldmann and Geisbert (2012) classified EVD as a classical zoonosis disease. Despite the fact that EVD is transmitted from non-human primates to humans, the natural reservoir of EVD is still unknown (CDC, 2014; Jones, 2011). In keeping with Feldmann and Geisbert (2012), several studies were conducted to identify the natural reservoir of EVD. These studies confirmed that some bats infected experimentally with EVD do not die, thus confirming the possibility that bats may be the natural reservoirs of EVD. WHO (2014) confirmed the studies that African fruit bats of the Pteropodidae family may be the natural reservoir for EVD. While this may be true, human-to-human transmission is most critical and the need to contain the spread of the EVD remains a global challenge (Feldmann & Geisbert, 2012).

Jones (2011) and WHO (2014) described EVD and Marburg viruses to be the only filoviruses that cause severe hemorrhagic fever syndrome in humans and non-human primates such as monkeys and chimpanzees. The CDC (2014) noted that EVD is an infrequent and fatal illness reportable to the National Notifiable Disease Surveillance System (NNDSS) throughout the United States and its territories. The CDC (2014) concurred with WHO (2014) that early recognition of EVD is critical for infection control. People coming into the United States from any EVD declared country should notify health care providers. Doctors and nurses should evaluate any patient suspected or displaying symptoms of EVD. The CDC (2014) classified a suspected EVD patient as a Person Under Investigation (PUI). A PUI should have consistent symptoms and risk factors such: as elevated body temperature or subjective fever or symptoms, including a severe headache, fatigue, muscle pain, vomiting, diarrhea, abdominal pain, or unexplained hemorrhage (CDC, 2014).

SEASONAL OUTBREAKS OF EBOLA VIRUS DISEASE

According to Leroy et al. (2005), most EVD outbreaks have usually occurred during the rainy season or at the beginning of the dry season. In West Africa especially Liberia, the rainy season runs from mid-May to the end of September, whilst the dry season begins from mid-October to the end of April. During the dry season, fruit bats believed to be the natural reservoir of Ebola begin to give birth; and at this time (dry season) fruits become scarce in the forest. The scarcity of forest fruits due to the seasonal variations and the concomitant increase in the ape and bat populations result in competition for fruit during these periods, thus creating conditions for a closer and increased contact. It is this increased contact between the naturally infected fruit bats and apes that could influence the contact with animals thus leading to Ebola outbreaks in human populations for similar reasons (Leroy et al. 2005). Most of the previous and the 2014 EVD outbreaks occurred in villages where individuals rely on the forest for food and animal skins for costumes. The EVD then makes its way into towns and cities through infected-human migration (trade) or family visitations.

THE ROLE OF MEDIA DURING EPIDEMICS

According to the International Federation of Red Cross and Red Crescent Societies (IFRC & RCS, 2012), the 2000-2001 EVD outbreak in Gulu, Uganda was significantly contained with the help of social mobilization. De Roo et al. (1995) confirmed that EVD awareness and education through the media or local cultural performances (drama groups) designed to win the confidence and support of rural residents must first be put into effect while awaiting the invention of EVD vaccines and or cure. The effective use of media such as radio stations educating communities through local dialects about EVD can prove to be successful (IFRC & RCS, 2012). The use of community drama groups demonstrating EVD-related messages is critical to fighting ostracism and stigma associated with EVD.

WHO (2014) agreed that the use of media including documentary films will enhance epidemic preparedness and response. The extensive circulation of education banners, posters, and flyers bearing guidelines that emphasize stopping of traditional and social practices such as handshakes, public or large gatherings, indigenous healing practices as well as cultural burial rituals is pivotal to containing EVD (WHO, 2014). The IFRC & RCS (2012) recounted the role of the media during the 2000-2001 EVD outbreaks in Gulu, Uganda. The media role helped trained healthcare workers and community resource individuals to participate in EVD surveillance. This approach of the epidemic response was relevant because it helped to create an effective collective management response effort through multisectoral collaboration (IFRC & RCS, 2012).

The epidemic control efforts through media also consisted of trained volunteers disseminating EVD-related messages in affected areas. The volunteers carried out health promotion and media campaigns to include a house-to-house contact tracings and follow-ups. Some volunteers were trained counselors and offered psychosocial support and rehabilitation services. Others were involved in the distribution of non-food items to discharged survivors and their families. Training was provided to locals in epidemic control and prevention (IFRC & RCS, 2012). Jones (2011) added that the initial outbreaks of EVD in 1976 received virtually no media coverage, and western concern regarding EVD was very low. Jones (2011) recounted that in 1989, EVD was detected in a shipment of crab-eating macaque monkeys to a laboratory in Reston, Virginia. The role of media, in the Reston case, was limited and or not effective.

According to Chowell and Nishiura (2014), the 2014 EVD outbreaks in West Africa created another opportunity for healthcare workers and policy makers to improve the role of media during epidemic outbreaks. An effective media campaign should first be put in place to help misinformed communities understand the cause of EVD and persuade community members to work along with healthcare workers to combat the disease. This will help to take away the stigma of fear for community members who see isolation centers as a death sentence for their sick relatives (Chowell & Nishiura, 2014).

The global community has been criticized for not rapidly responding to EVD since its introduction in 1976 and until the 2014 West Africa outbreaks (Jones, 2011). Lamontagne et al. (2014) interjected that since the initial outbreak of EVD in 1976, the role of developed countries in finding a cure and establishing effective control mechanism has been sluggish. EVD phenomenon is a tragic validation of the cliché that the world has become a global village in which what happens in one village in most cases may rapidly affect another either for good or bad. European countries and the United States only actively got involved when citizens of their respective countries working in EVD-affected countries such as Liberia were tested positive with EVD (Lamontagne et al., 2014). Jones (2011) concurred with Lamontagne et al. (2014) and stressed that there is a need to aggressively promote media coverage of EVD presence in any part of the world and pursue the improvement of health centers and make available necessary supplies, training, and education in these affected regions as means to eradicate EVD (Jones, 2011).

CURRENT HEALTHCARE AND POLICY INITIATIVES

Due to the poor health infrastructure of the affected West African countries, coupled with the global challenge of finding a cure or appropriate preventative measures to contain EVD, the disease is far from containment (Gomes et al., 2014). As described by Gomes et al. (2014), the current intervention strategies put together to contain EVD has proven not to be effective in the wake of social and traditional practices combined with poor governments' policies. Gomes et al. (2014) emphasized that in West Africa and Liberia in particular, cultural, economic, and political factors have hampered the effectiveness of the intervention strategies used by local and international health practitioners. The lack of laboratory capacity, and equipped quarantining centers and the lack of or ignoring the use of PPE helped to exposed health workers and the general public to EVD.

Tambo (2014) stressed that funding efforts for containing and preventing the spread of EVD in West Africa and Africa as a whole should be encouraged. Gomes et al. (2014) concurred with Tambo (2014) that funding for the improvement of medical programs or facilities in West Africa and Africa as a whole should be encouraged but inserted that these governments' officials are corrupt, and fear that the funds may be diverted into their person benefits. Gomes et al. (2014) stressed that institutions such as the World Bank, the International Monetary Fund (IMF), and the WHO, among others have over several decades contributed to the improvement of health care in Africa, yet health care conditions remain deplorable. WHO (2015) concurred with Gomes et al. (2014) and added that these governments should change their current policies that impede the improvement of their respective health care systems. Tambo (2014) added that some of the current health care policies on books in these West African countries are good but lacks implementation. Those in charge of enforcing these policies are themselves corrupt, thus leaving impoverished communities the fund is intended to benefit. Every EVD outbreak has come with challenges based on its geographical location to include culture, traditions, and beliefs.

Tambo (2014) identified five of the many challenges healthcare providers and policymakers may incur when responding to EVD outbreaks:

- The inadequacy in developing and implementing a surveillance-response system against EVD in Africa.
- The lack of community education and their knowledge about EVD outbreak which triggers panic, anxiety, psychosocial trauma, isolation, and dignity; engendering stigma, community ostracism and resistance to associated cultural factors and public health consequences.
- The lack of financial resources and trained healthcare workers
- Weak community and national health system operational plans for prevention and control responses, practices and management.
- The lack of leadership and coordination including the development of new strategies, tools, and approaches, such as improved diagnostics and therapies including vaccines which can assist in preventing, controlling and containing EVD outbreaks as well as the spread of the disease.

Tambo (2014) suggested that healthcare practitioners and policymakers can work to improve upon the above challenges which will set standards for approaching future EVD outbreaks (Tambo, 2014).

GAPS IN THE STUDY

Most of the literature reviewed and selected to support this study largely focused on factors for the spread and transmission of EVD. However, a little or no research has yet described how people are coping with the threat of EVD, thereby creating a gap that needs to be addressed. In this direction, according to WHO (2015), it is crucial to identify and understand how survivors, family caregivers, and the general public experience coping with the threat of EVD. Significant questions this study explored include; how survivors and family caregivers perceived the disease, their reactions, and their experience of coping with the threat and uncertainty of EVD.

WHO (2015) further explained that the consequence of a life threatening disease and its treatment or sequela has a significant effect on the life of the affected person; this may include their physical appearance and their psychological perception of themselves. In this situation, the issue of self-concept becomes critical because of their physical change or self-image. Living with the

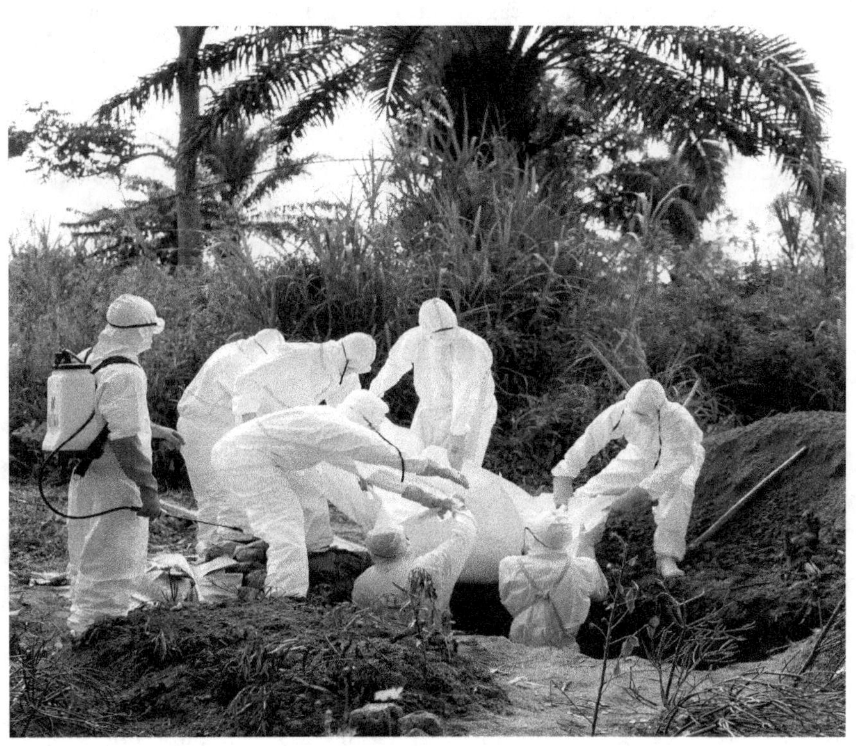

Burial of Ebola Victim
Courtesy of Augustine Manneh Sumo

physical change the disease may have inflicted on the survivors, may cause feelings of inferiority and low self-esteem thereby affecting their well-being (WHO, 2015). This study is designed to understand how EVD survivors and family caregivers coped under the threat of EVD.

Farmer (2001) agreed that combining survivors difficulty in adjusting to an altered body image is the fear of how will the community react to their altered appearance. In most cases, survivors may shy away from others in their community fearing that they will be considered less than human. It is against this background that this study investigated the overwhelming shame and embarrassment that may cause survivors to absent themselves and withdraw from social activities. In school going adolescents, such stigmatization may result to dropping out of school. WHO (2015) on the other hand argued that survivors, family caregivers, and the general public could develop resentment toward their governments based on bad policies or decrees that did not address their interest. A significant negative consequence survivors may have to deal with are those traumatic experiences according to WHO (2015).

As part of their experiences, the post-traumatic stress that survivors struggled to overcome was also explored. It is believed that survivors may try to avoid situations related to their situation, thus becoming hysterical and fearful about activities that remind them of the hurtful experience (WHO, 2015). Investigating the social economic implications of individuals coping in the shadows of a life-threatening disease such as EVD could fill in a gap of scholarly contribution related to EVD, more so to the fear and panic, it creates in communities. Despite all the good containment techniques recommended or previously applied in past and the 2014 EVD outbreaks in West Africa, it is crucial that a good understanding of the public's perspectives regarding EVD is designed through community full participation. Doing so would help in demystifying and reducing the fear and panic associated with EVD (WHO, 2015). This study also investigated if by educating at-risk populations using perspectives that incorporate their own understanding and beliefs about EVD could likely result in better epidemic control (WHO, 2015).

SUMMARY

The purpose of this literature review was to examine the main issues related to EVD including the economic, poverty, policy, cultural, and social factors that influenced EVD outbreaks, especially the 2014 EVD event in West Africa. The 2014 EVD outbreaks in Guinea, Liberia, and Sierra Leone were initially transmitted through human-animal contact. The literature reviewed noted that EVD is not an airborne disease; it can be spread through human-human contact with bodily fluids of infected persons. The stigma survivors experienced on a day-to-day basis was highlighted. Generally, Chapter 2 discussed in details the main issues related to the spread of EVD, including the policies initiated by government intended to contain EVD. Past intervention techniques to contain EVD was also discussed in the literature review and recommendations made to contain the spread of EVD.

Chapter 3 focused on methods and procedures and once more discussed the purpose of the study. Sections in Chapter 3 include the research design which cited the strengths and weaknesses and focused on issues of internal and external validity of the design. Chapter 3 highlighted the target population and the selection of research participants and the method of sampling. Chapter 3 further detailed the procedures for conducting the study including informed consent protocols for human participants, and data collection instruments. The research questions were once more stated in the proper form and style. Chapter 3 further described the data collection analysis procedures including data coding and expected findings.

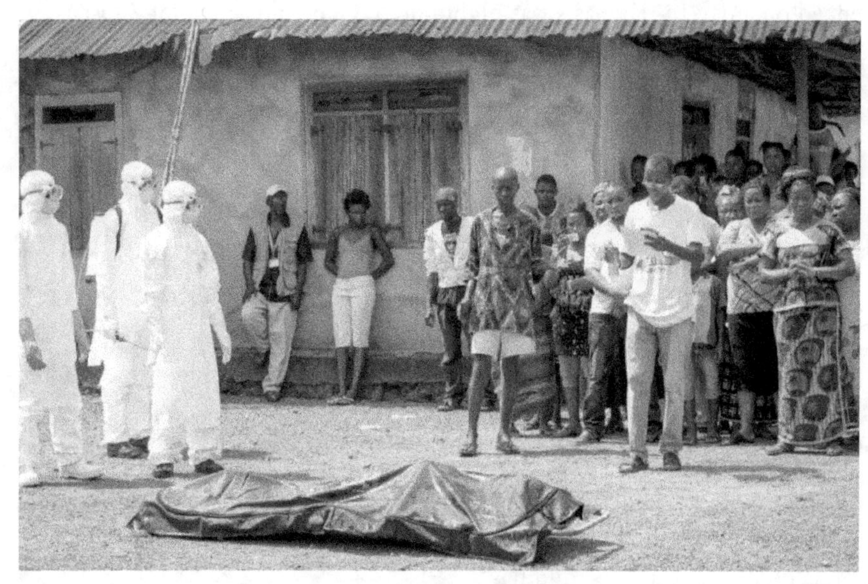

A Dead Victim of Ebola Virus Disease abandoned in the street
Courtesy of Augustine Manneh Sumo

CHAPTER 3

RESEARCH METHOD

INTRODUCTION

This chapter described the research method employed for this study. I also described the research design and rationale, the role I played as the researcher, the selected research participants, and the instruments I used to conduct this study. Additionally, this chapter discussed procedures related to recruitment and participation, data collection, and data analysis, and as well as issues of trustworthiness and ethical procedures.

In this this study, I addressed the social, economic, and policy factors that contributed to the spread of the 2014 EVD outbreak in Liberia. I also examined how residents of Monrovia coped with the threat of EVD and its effect on survivors, family caregivers, and the general public. Primarily, the study focused on EVD survivors and their family caregivers. Another point of focus is that the Liberian government was ill-equipped to efficiently contain the 2014 EVD outbreak due to inadequate training for hospitals and healthcare workers. The Liberian government's mandatory cremation policies and the banning of public gatherings further exacerbated the spread of EVD. WHO (2014) noted that during the first 6 months of EVD outbreak, 10,666 individuals were infected and 4,808 died. WHO (2015) further confirmed that 375 health workers were infected and 189 died. Over 60% of the overall EVD infection and mortality occurred in the city of Monrovia.

RESEARCH DESIGN AND RATIONALE

This qualitative case study primarily involved inputs from EVD survivors and their family caregivers. I also solicited inputs from government policy makers (government officials), NGO staff, academicians, and reporters from the media to answer the research questions and draw a conclusion from the study. I identified these individuals because they provided care and other services to EVD patients during the 2014 EVD outbreak. Official letters of invitation were sent to them to participate in the study. Flyers bearing the researcher's phone number and physical contact address were developed and posted in conspicuous locations in the city of Monrovia inviting reporters from the media and academicians to also participate in the study. Upon signing up, official letters of invitation were sent to them to participate in the study. By using a case study design, this study explored the social, economic, and policy factors that contributed to the spread of the 2014 EVD outbreak in Monrovia (WHO, 2015). I recruited 10 EVD survivors and 10 family caregivers in the three selected communities while the other 10 participants included government officials, NGO staff, academicians, and reporters from the media. The interviews consisted of open-ended questions in the semi-structure form and were tape-recorded for transcription and analysis. In this regard, the following research questions were selected to answer the goal of the study:

RQ1: How did survivors and family caregivers cope with the threat of EVD in Monrovia in 2014?

RQ2: What social, cultural, and economic factors may have contributed to the spread of EVD in Monrovia in 2014?

RQ3: How did government policies of mandatory cremation and banning of public gatherings affect the containment of EVD in Monrovia in 2014?

RQ4: What social stigma did EVD cause among survivors?

Yin (2014) states that a research design is a logical sequence that connects the empirical data to the research questions of the study, and subsequently to its conclusion. This process as Yin (2014) explained can move the researcher from a broad philosophy and theoretical perspective to the validation of the study.

Case study research as defined by Merriam (2009) involves an empirical inquiry that examines a contemporary phenomenon in-depth within its real life context, particularly in cases when the boundaries between phenomenon and context are not clearly evident. This case study query could lead to some distinctive situations to discover new variables that the current data has not identified. This could strengthen the evidence-base of the study through multiple resources converging in a triangulation fashion that can benefit the study (Merriam, 2009).

The research design utilized resources such as documents, archival records, interviews, and observations of participants to build the understanding of the experiences of research participants by use of the case study approach. The Yin theory supports researchers by providing a simple explanation of the observed relations relevant to the phenomenon. McMillian and Schumacher (2001) gave a supporting explanation as it relates to the principles of data collection. McMillian and Schumacher (2001) explained that the Yin theory uses multiple sources of evidence (triangulation) to build converging lines of inquiry and strengthen construct validity, thereby maintaining a chain of evidence.

In regard to emphasizing specific boundaries and the use of multiple data sources, a case study inquiry for this study included the following characteristics; (a) it focused on the "why" and "how" questions of the study, (b) it did not influence the behavior of research participants or those involved, and (c) it was advantageous to examine contextual conditions because they were believed to be relevant to the study (Yin, 2014). Therefore, understanding the impact cannot be investigated appropriately outside the boundaries of those that experience the phenomenon. Additionally, the use of multiple data sources provided a broader and richer picture of the case. With the permission and consent from participants, I conducted interviews in participants' homes, offices of government officials, NGO's conference rooms, and community centers. This allowed for a face-to-face interaction with participants that built a working rapport and created an atmosphere of cooperation and collaboration, which led to follow-up interviews. The data collection process involved responses obtained from participants through interviews while guaranteeing participants of their confidentiality. In this manner, in-depth, context-rich responses from participants were obtained. In the context of McMillan and Schumacher (2001), I observed participants' behaviors as it relates to EVD stigma. This process created the atmosphere of actually understanding the participants' emotions relating to the phenomenon. Accordingly, I recorded field notes based on specific criteria for collecting data during the observation of participants. Relating to data analysis and interpretation, I kept an active journal for the purpose of reflecting on potential biases and assumptions including decisions. These procedures ensured strategies that enhanced trustworthiness for this study.

The decision to conduct this study on inputs from EVD survivors, their family caregivers, government officials, NGO staff, academicians, and reporters from the media in three selected communities in Monrovia was based on the assumption that individuals in the selected communities reflect the demographic characteristics and experiences with the outbreak of the entire city of Monrovia. These individuals shared the same values, culture, beliefs and standards, and the reaction of one could represent the others. The design choice for this study was driven by personal values and beliefs. Yin (2014) stated that philosophical assumptions designed to guide a research should be based on the followings: an attitude toward the nature of reality (ontology), including how the investigator understands what she or he understands (epistemology), taking into account the research values (axiology), the appropriate research language (rhetoric), and the method to be used in the process (methodology).

The framework mentioned above highlighted the human motivation and behavior side of this study. This is critical to the study because in situations such as epidemics; people react to the situation based on what they have previously learned or inherited (culture) and believed (values) (Bandura, 1997). The Bandura SCT framework employed for this study suggested a theory of human motivation and action from a social cognitive perspective. In the SCT framework, Bandura (1997) stressed that the application of observational learning, imitation and modeling integrates a continuous interaction between behaviors, personal factors, cognition, and the environment. Behavior as Bandura (1997) explained refers to the complexity and skills, among others, related to an individual. The environment refers to where the phenomenon occurred and it describes the situation, roles, models, and the relationships. A personal factor (person) refers to cognition which describes self-efficacy, motives, and personality. The SCT as the guiding theoretical framework for this study was applied throughout this research.

ROLE OF THE RESEARCHER

Data collection, analysis, and interpretation of this study were the sole responsibility of the researcher. In this role, it was assumed that researcher biases could exist. In this regard, I used several strategies to limit bias such as asking quality questions, recognizing potential sources of biases, and remaining focused on the research goals (Patton, 2001) as means of addressing such biases throughout the study. I achieved this goal by recording comprehensive field notes that included reflection and subjectivity. It was crucial for the investigator to consider "self" as a researcher and "self" as it relates to the research topic as a precondition for handling potential biases during the study (Patton, 2001). Merriam (2009) explained that in a case study research study, it is significant for the researcher to investigate their own ideas and experiences with the phenomenon in question. Since there are broad philosophical assumptions, as explained by Patton (2001), the researcher should try to identify their personal assumptions before initiating the research study.

I used my personal perspective to investigate how Monrovians coped with the threat of EVD. As a public health practitioner and a public policy expert, I have witnessed several events such as epidemics that negatively affected communities due to the lack of appropriate staff training, low-quality resources, and policies. During these episodes, I have never fully understood the experiences of community members who experience the phenomenon except for reporting the event. Through this research study, I was given the opportunity to explore the human experience side of the 2014 EVD outbreak in Monrovia. In this role, I suspended any personal understanding of the phenomenon so that a true and accurate interpretation of the event can be implemented. I am presently working as the Director for a nonprofit organization catering to children who suffer from sickle cell disease (SCD). I am not affiliated with WHO, similar organizations, or have any form of relationship with the participants for this study, even though I am a citizen of Liberia and a former resident of Monrovia.

RESEARCH METHOD

I used a qualitative research method that explored the lived experiences of EVD survivors and their family caregivers in Monrovia. McMillan and Schumacher

(2001) stated that qualitative research method is a descriptive research that seeks to understand the how, who, and what of phenomena. Additionally, Yin (2014) stated that researchers should use qualitative research method to study individual cases with an absence of general regularities in social contexts. Merriam (2009) pointed out that a qualitative research method helps to determine how individuals or groups draw conclusions about social or human experiences. The qualitative research method is flexible because it gives room to the researcher to amend the interview as it progresses. It also allows researchers to incorporate unexpected findings that help to understand the research problem. Qualitative research methodology adopts semi-structured questions to elicit conversation about the lived experiences of the participants (Merriam, 2009). The qualitative research methodology allows the researcher to participate first-hand in the data collection process. Further, the qualitative research method is suitable for events where the number and type of observations available do not readily lend themselves to consistent measurement and statistical analysis.

SELECTION OF RESEARCH PARTICIPANTS

Participants for this case study were primarily EVD survivors along with their family caregivers, officials of government, NGO staff, academicians, and reporters from the media in three selected communities in the city of Monrovia. The three selected communities were the hardest hit by the 2014 EVD outbreak in Monrovia. I recruited 30 participants which included 10 EVD survivors, 10 family caregivers to participate in the study. The 10 EVD survivors and 10 family caregivers directly experienced the impact of EVD. Therefore, their input supported the study to achieve its goal. I also recruited 10 participants including government officials, NGO staff, academicians, and reporters from the media to support the study achieve data saturation. These additional participants were individuals who provided care and other services for EVD patients during the 2014 EVD outbreak. According to Bertaux (1981), 15 is the smallest acceptable sample size in all qualitative research. Charmaz (2006) argued that the aims of the study are the ultimate driver of the project design, and the sample size. Since most Liberians share a lot in common such as culture and tradition, it is assumed that residents of the three selected communities will reflect the demographic characteristics and experiences with the outbreak.

The selection process of research participants for this study began with the researcher writing a formal letter of collaboration to institutions in Monrovia where EVD patients and their contacts including family caregivers were isolated and treated. These institutions include the Ministry of Health and Social Welfare of Liberia, the Liberia National Red Cross, and Médecins Sans Frontières. The above-mentioned institutions agreed in advance to support the study. Therefore, based on the list of EVD survivors and their family caregiver provided by the above institutions, I selected 10 participants of EVD survivors and 10 family caregivers based on the inclusion criteria guiding the study. Subsequently, I made phone calls and also in-person contacts with participants and invited them to the study. The other 10 potential participants included government officials (from the Ministry of Health and Social Welfare of Liberia), NGO staff (from Médecins Sans Frontières), and (Liberia National Red Cross), academicians, and reporters from the media (from the city of Monrovia). These individuals provided care and other services to EVD patients during the 2014 EVD outbreak. Participants from the above-mentioned institutions received official letters of invitation to participate in the study. Flyers bearing the researcher's phone number and physical contact address were developed and posted in conspicuous locations in the city of Monrovia inviting reporters from the media and academicians to also participate in the study. Upon signing up, official letters of invitation were also sent to them to participate in the study.

SAMPLING PROCEDURES

Additional potential participants were selected based on the snowball sampling criteria suggested by Patton (2001). Patton (2001) stated that when conducting sampling, the investigator should employ a sampling technique that will lead to a careful selection of participants depending on the informational needs and inclusion criteria. Participants were selected based on the following inclusion criteria: (a) participants must be an adult 18 years and above, (b) participants must be an EVD survivor or family caregiver who lived in Monrovia during and after the 2014 EVD outbreak, (c) participants must be a member from the media who covered the event, (d) participants must be an official of government or NGO staff who provided care and services to EVD survivors and (e) participants must be willing to participate in the interview process without any monetary compensation. Participants were selected without regard to gender, race, and religion.

For the purpose of data saturation, a snowball sampling technique was chosen to support the researcher achieve the goal of this study. Snowball sampling helps a researcher to draw conclusions for the entire population after conducting a study on samples taken from the same population. According to Biernacki and Waldorf (1981), data saturation occurs at a point where the same answer keeps appearing with little or no variation in many interviews. Biernacki and Waldorf (1981) further argued that data saturation is achieved when the researcher obtains all relevant information on a phenomenon. For this study, 30 participants were selected in three communities that were the hardest hit by the 2014 EVD in Monrovia. At least 20 of the 30 research participants were EVD survivors and their family caregivers in each of the three communities; while the other 10 participants included government officials, NGO staff, academicians, and reporters from the media. The interviews consisted of open-ended questions in the semi-structure form and were tape-recorded for transcription and analysis. The face-to-face interviews were conducted either at the participants' home or at an agreed upon community center. The interviews were composed of 10 to 15 questions and each interview lasted between 45 minutes to one hour. The sampling process for this study began after Walden's IRB approved the study.

INSTRUMENTATION

The primary instrument for data collection for this case study was an interview. An interview helps the researcher to observe verbal and non-verbal signs and conduct documentation. The process also helps the researcher to build rapport with research participants in a more cordial manner (McMillan & Schumacher, 2001). The instrument (interview) comprised of 10-15 open-ended interview questions developed by the researcher, while maintaining direct focus on the phenomenon being examined. The interview questions were focused primarily on values, beliefs, and experiences community members share as it relates to EVD.

Two experts in Monrovia who are knowledgeable in the field of research and especially who helped to treat survivors of the 2014 EVD outbreak initially validated the interview questions for content and standards. This professional evaluation of the research questions increased the likelihood of focus and alignment to achieve desire research goal. The interview questions were based on McMillan and Schumacher (2001) suggestions for conducting effective qualitative research interviews. These interview questions focused primarily on the values and beliefs the community members share as it relates to disease and illness, specifically, EVD and the contributions community members can make to stop the spread and transmission of EVD when an outbreak occur.

Another technique for data collection for this case study was observation. The observation technique helped to collect data during interactions such as interviews with selected participants. These interactions were in the form of group meetings (field work) for the purpose of group interviews, observations and documentation (triangulation). Participants were observed specifically, their emotion, passion, consistency, and compatibility in their respective responses. These group meetings were conducted in a natural setting using the criteria suggested by McMillan and Schumacher (2001) as follows: (a) the physical setting of their homes, and (b) public facilities such as a library or community center. The technique of observation allowed the researcher to record field notes and reflections.

RECRUITMENT PROCEDURES

Upon the IRB approval, I started the recruitment process of research participants for this study by making phone calls. Participants were also contacted in person. I sent letters of invitation to individuals according to records of the below listed institutions: The Ministry of Health and Social Welfare of Liberia, the Liberia National Red Cross, and Médecins Sans Frontières. Participants were then selected from the list of adult EVD survivors and family caregivers based on records from the above institutions. Subsequently, I made phone calls and made in-person contact with participants and invited them to the study.

The snowball sampling procedure was used to recruit other participants such as government officials (from the Ministry of Health and Social Welfare of Liberia) and NGO staff (from Médecins Sans Frontières and Liberia

National Red Cross). Flyers bearing the researcher's phone number and physical contact was developed and posted in conspicuous locations in the city of Monrovia inviting members of the media and academicians to participate in the study. As stated before, the issue with Ebola in Liberia is very crucial, so every institution or individual was willing to cooperate in helping find a controlled mechanism for the containment of the virus and or cure. The above mentioned institutions agreed in advance to support the study by providing contact information of EVD survivors and their family caregivers whom they provided care and treatment during the 2014 EVD outbreak.

DATA COLLECTION PROCEDURES

Before any data were collected for this study, a consent form application was first filed with the IRB requesting authorization to conduct this study. Data collection began after the IRB approved the study. The data collection process for this study included interviews, observations, and documentation of EVD survivors and their family caregivers. Data collection also included interviews of officials of government from the Ministry of Health and Social Welfare of Liberia, NGO staff from the Liberia National Red Cross, Médecins Sans Frontières, academicians and members from the media. Concerning collecting data from EVD survivors, interviews was conducted in the following locations based on participant preference: in participants' homes, public library, and community center. Interviews of government officials, NGO staff, academicians and members of the media were done in their respective offices and conference rooms. With the consent of participants, I tape-recorded the interviews. A notebook was used to take notes and to make reflections to responses. Before the interview, I told participants that they can stop the interview at any time once they feel uncomfortable to continue the process. Upon request, participants received copy of the interview script. At the end of each interview, I thanked participants for their participation and informed them that they may be called upon again if necessary for follow-up interviews. I initially assured all participants of the confidentiality of their information and participation.

In addition to information gathered during interviews, I also observed participants during the study in order to gain understanding of their physical and emotional reactions to questions. Each meeting or interview time varied

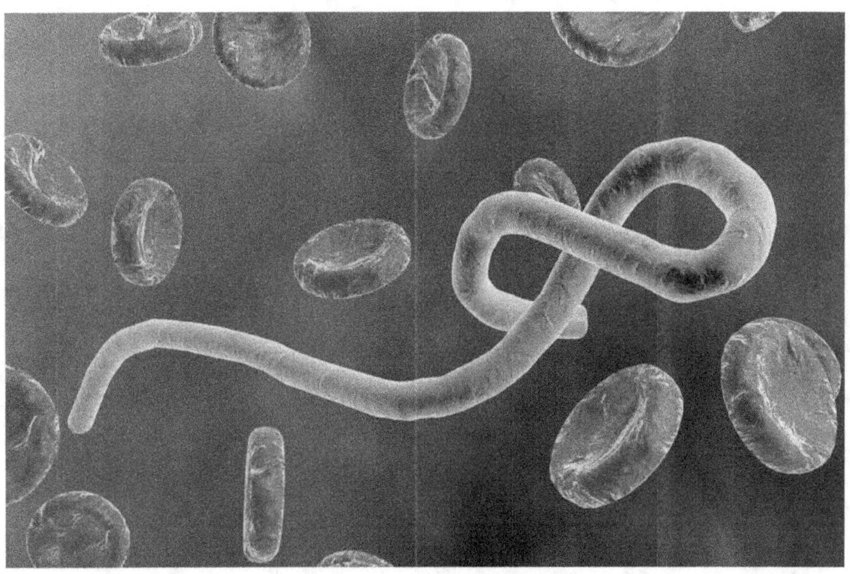

Marburg and Ebola Virus Disease

The related Marburg virus, genus Marburgvirus, is morphologically indistinguishable and induces symptoms similar to Ebolavirus.

Marburg virus disease is a highly virulent disease that causes haemorrhagic fever, with a fatality ratio of up to 88%. It is in the same family as the virus that causes Ebola virus disease. Two large outbreaks that occurred simultaneously in Marburg and Frankfurt in Germany, and in Belgrade, Serbia, in 1967, led to the initial recognition of the disease. The outbreak was associated with laboratory work using African green monkeys imported from Uganda.

Courtesy of World Health Organization

between 45 minutes to one hour. During this time of observation, an observation data collection form which was developed and evaluated by professionals. The observation data collection form was used to record field notes and research reflections in accordance with McMillan and Schumacher (2001) recommendation for observation. During the process of interviews and observations, I solicited document accounts about the participants' lived experiences as they relate to EVD, such as diary accounts of their day-to-day experiences coping with the threat of EVD. Available public documents such as newspapers, newsletters, and online blogs relating to the lived experiences of individuals who survived EVD were also reviewed.

DATA ANALYSIS PLAN

As stated earlier, I collected data through in-depth face-to-face interviews and observations of participants. I also solicited document accounts about the participants' lived experiences as they relate to EVD. Such documents included diary accounts of the day-to-day experiences of coping with the threat of EVD. I also attempted to solicit any available public records such as newspapers, newsletters, and online blogs relating to the lived experiences of individuals who survived the 2014 EVD for reviewed.

Data analysis for this qualitative study was based on configuring collected data into comprehensible information (Merriam, 2009). The data analysis process occurred throughout the duration of this study. I employed the use of NVivo 10 to manage, organize, and keep track of data. These included raw data such as interviews, questionnaires, observations, and audio recordings.

Two steps were required to accomplish this goal. In the first step, using NVivo 10 software, interview data was transcribed and categorized by establishing codes. I ensured that the interview transcripts were read through and recordings listened to thus creating the opportunity to make marginal notes. This process supported the theory of using the line-by-line coding according to Yin (2014) recommendations for qualitative research. In this regard, I followed the exact procedures when the observation field notes and reflections were analyzed. NVivo 10 ensured a content analysis process for all documents.

In the second step, NVivo 10 was utilized to initiate themes or patterns. Accordingly, the themes and disparities that transpired from the coded and categorized data determined the key findings. These were analyzed in relation to the central and related research questions for the study and interpreted according to the theoretical framework and the literature review.

TRUSTWORTHINESS

The standards of trustworthiness and quality for this study were emphasized on the concepts of credibility, validity, transferability, dependability, and confirmability through the reporting of research findings. Research quality is when the research work conforms to the methodology of the study (Yin, 2014). To ensure trustworthiness Lincoln and Guba (1985) stated that the researcher must demonstrate that transition from raw data to informed data is valid. Trustworthiness can be achieved in a study when there is confidence in the truth (credibility) of the findings, and that the findings should have applicability (transferability) in other contexts. Further, trustworthiness according to Lincoln and Guba (1985), ensures the findings are consistent (dependability) and could be repeated, and can demonstrate a degree of neutrality (confirmability) in a manner in which the results of the study are shaped by the respondents and not researcher bias, motivation, or interest.

CREDIBILITY

Qualitative research credibility relates to the internal validity of the study, particularly, the way the research findings should match the reality. In quantitative research, the formation of credibility parallels with the criterion of validity in order to ensure that the researcher reports exactly what took place and not what the researcher expect to take place (Yin, 2014). Additionally, in qualitative research, credibility requires that data reported must support the findings. Merriam (2009) stated that the findings should portray an exact description of the experiences of those who experienced the phenomenon so that people who have shared the same experience can easily recognize and find it believable.

Merriam (2009) recommended that qualitative researchers should use the following strategies to improve the credibility of the study: (a) triangulation, (b) members checks, (c) and adequate engagement during data collection, (d) reflexivity, and (e) peer-review. This study primarily focused on the triangulation strategy that was utilized the in-depth interviews, observations and documentation for data collection. The triangulation strategy according to Merriam (2009) uses multiple methods, data sources, investigators, and theories to confirm emerging findings. The triangulation strategy triangulated data by comparing and cross-checking data sources, which included interviews, observations, and documentation to confirm the conclusions of the study. The member checks strategy was intended to assist the researcher to improve the credibility of the study by presenting the negative instances or discrepant findings that challenged any emerging findings, was not used. The member checks strategy (Merriam, 2009), should have also allow the researcher to query participants as means to determine if the tentative findings of this study are credible.

Adequate time was spent with participants as means of engaging them in meaningful discussions about their experiences with EVD with focus on seeking discrepant and negative cases. This process maximized saturation of data. The reflexivity strategy (Merriam, 2009) allowed the researcher to conduct critical self-reflection regarding assumptions, worldviews, biases, theoretical orientation, and relationship to the study that could have affected the investigation. The peer-review strategy which was also not used in this study   involved reviewing related scholarly articles and discussions with colleagues regarding the procedures of the study, the consistency of emerging findings with the raw data, and tentative interpretation.

TRANSFERABILITY

Yin (2014) defined transferability as the external validity to which the findings of one study is applicable to others. Yin further stated that the representation of samples is not a determinant of transferability in qualitative research, it depends on how well the study allow for the reader to deduce whether similar processes and methods will relate to their own settings. I used the rich thick description recommended by Merriam (2009) to improve the transferability of this qualitative study. This strategy presented the setting and findings of the study and helped to implement the maximum variation of the typical sample. Additionally, the rich thick strategy also presented the participants, the data analysis procedures, and the findings. A rich thick strategy provides sufficient description to conceptualize the study. In this regard, the typicality of the sample for EVD survivors and family caregivers in the communities this study selected was typical of the many communities that were hit by the EVD outbreak in Monrovia.

DEPENDABILITY

Merriam (2009) referred to dependability in qualitative research as reliability or consistency to the extent that research findings can be generalized. In this direction, Merriam (2009) suggests that the strategies of triangulation, peer-review, reflexivity, and an audit trail can improve the dependability of a qualitative study. An audit trail, in this case study, presented a detailed account of the methods, procedures, and decisions for the study. All processes of this research were consistent with the philosophical and methodological principles of a case study research.

CONFIRMABILITY

In qualitative research, the perception of confirmability correlates with the idea of objectivity. I provided findings that met the goal of the study, not the result of the biases and subjectivity of the researcher (Merriam, 2009). The strategy of triangulation was used to improve the objectivity of the study. This was done by constantly cross-checking data sources during analysis of the data. To assure the objectivity of this study, the strategy of reflexivity was also applied to assure that the data collected and analyzed represented the experiences, views, and beliefs of the participants, not the researcher.

Reflexivity, as defined by Merriam (2009), is the way to reflect critically on oneself as a researcher. During qualitative research, potential bias must be realized immediately and corrected to enable the researcher to present an honest report thus avoiding subjectivity. This study was designed to maintain a log in which the personal beliefs and assumptions of the researcher was documented for the purpose of clarifications and reflections. Subjectivity and bias were minimized by applying strict protocols during data collection and analysis. Decisions made in this study were objective as possible and that all findings were addressed through reflective commentary according to the log being maintained.

ETHICAL PROCEDURES

Ethics is the study of what is right and wrong and the way people ought to live (Patton, 2001). Trustworthiness in qualitative research is contingent on the ethics of the researcher (Merriam, 2009). For this study, the IRB guidelines supported by Walden University in order to be responsive to ethical considerations through all stages of the study were followed. Primarily, data for this study came from in-depth interviews with EVD survivors and their family caregiver, government officials, NGO staff, academicians, and reporters from the media. Therefore, before initiating any interview, a consent form designed for the purpose of informed consent was filled in and signed by the interviewee thus authorizing the interview. The consent form was the agreement between the researcher and the research participant and clearly stated that all information provided will be treated confidentially. Research participants were informed beforehand that the interview will be taped recorded. Generally, before the interviews, participants were assured of the strictest confidence to their privacy and responses. The researcher obtained and store data in the following formats: Paper (journal), electronic (computer), or audio (tape-recorder). Data were protected using a locked file cabinet for papers and a password protected computer and flash drive (thumb). The researcher ensured full security precautions such as locked cabinets, computer or flash password protection. The researcher used codes instead of names on the interview document to ensure anonymity.

Another way this study addressed the issue of confidentiality was through the process of data cleaning (Howe et al., 2007). In this manner, identifiers were removed as means of creating a clean data set. The risk in this study refers to the fusion of the likelihood and enormity of some future harm that could impact participants (Merriam, 2009). This study was designed to conduct in-depth interviews on the topic of EVD. In this direction, participants were first made aware of the interview topic and they were recruited based on their ability and willingness to speak on such topic.

The Samaritan Purse is a nonprofit organization offering trauma counseling services to survivors of the 2014 EVD in Monrovia. In any case, when a participant should need counseling as a result of their participation in this study, the Samaritan Purse offered such services free of charge. In relation to

Walden's vision for positive social change, participants were told that this study may potentially help to prevent the spread and transmission of EVD whenever an outbreak occurs.

SUMMARY

Chapter 3 highlighted the research method that was used to conduct the study. Chapter 3 described the research design and methodology employed for this study. Chapter 3 also described the research design and rationale, and the research questions. Chapter 3 further highlighted the role of the researcher and explained how biases were handled. Other topics in this section include the research method, selection of research participants, sampling procedures, instrumentation, and recruitment procedures. The data collection procedure was also discussed including data analysis plan, trustworthiness, and credibility, transferability, dependability, and confirmability. Chapter 3 concluded by discussing the ethical procedures that guided this study and the introduction of Chapter 4. Chapter 4 focused primarily on the results of the study. This chapter discussed the setting of the study, research questions, demographics, data collection, data analysis, and evidence of trustworthiness.

CHAPTER 4

RESULTS

INTRODUCTION

The purpose of conducting this qualitative case study was to examine the experiences of EVD survivors, family caregivers, government officials, NGO staff, academicians, and members of the media as it relates to coping with the threat of Ebola. By using a case study design, I focused on individuals who directly or indirectly experience the 2014 EVD outbreak in Monrovia. I conducted interviews with EVD survivors, family caregivers, government officials, NGO staff, academicians, and members of the media to investigate what it takes to cope with the threat of Ebola. The research site included participants' homes, conference rooms of NGOs, offices of government officials, academicians, and reporters from the media. Participants were all adults, 18 years old and above. I selected EVD survivors and their family caregivers from three communities in Monrovia that were the hardest hit by EVD in 2014. I reviewed documents such as diaries from participants regarding their experiences with EVD during this study.

Central to creating the context of the study and addressing readers' comprehension is incorporating and providing study details. In this regard, Chapter 4 began with restating the research questions, pilot study, setting, and demographic information specific to the participants. Chapter 4 continued with the data collection and data analysis processes and details. Evidence of the study's trustworthiness represented through credibility, transferability, dependability, and confirmability, followed by the data collection and data analysis results. Details of the research questions findings, in support of Chapter 5 discussions, follow the presentation of the evidence of trustworthiness.

Chapter 4 then concluded with a summarized review of the presented information pertinent to the principle outcomes of the studied phenomenon.

RESEARCH QUESTIONS

The research questions for this study focused on the phenomenon of coping with the threat of EVD, including the social, cultural, and economic factors, social stigma, and governmental policies. The following questions were selected to answer the research goal:

RQ1: How did survivors and family caregivers cope with the threat of EVD in Monrovia in 2014?

RQ2: What social, cultural, and economic factors may have contributed to the spread of EVD in Monrovia in 2014?

RQ3: How did government policies of mandatory cremation and banning of public gathering affect the containment of EVD in Monrovia in 2014?

RQ4: What social stigma did EVD cause among survivors?

PILOT TEST

I conducted a pilot test for the interview preparation and implementation as stated by Archibald and Newman (2015). The pilot testing tested the interview questions on people who were similar to those who answered the actual interview questions. The pilot test assisted in determining if flaws, limitations, or other weaknesses existed within the interview design (Barth, Cook, Downs, Switzer, & Fischhoff, 2002). For example, the pilot participants helped the researcher understand areas potential participants understood or did not understand. I selected a total of 6 participants comprising 2 from each of the three selected communities that were the hardest hit by EVD for the pilot testing. I randomly selected these individuals to participate in the pilot study. I pilot tested the interview questions among the 6 members of the selected communities. These community members are currently living in these communities and were also living there during the EVD outbreak. The 6 selected community members are similar to the sample study population. After pilot testing the 6 participants with the one-on-one interview, each participant was asked to comment on any unclear or awkward questions.

Their responses were taken into account and some of the interview questions were revised accordingly.

I asked each participant to read and discuss any questions they had before signing the consent form (see Appendix B). For those who could not read, I read and explained to them details of the consent form and they acknowledged full understanding of the consent form. The recordings did not include the actual names of participants. Instead, participants were identified via coded combinations of letters and numbers developed by the researcher. Interview recordings were only accessible to the researcher and these were safely stored in a password protected computer and a locked cabinet. Interview transcripts were kept in a similar manner stored on a password protected computer and a locked cabinet that is only accessible to the researcher. Information that might have identified participants in any form was not recorded on the tapes nor included in the transcripts. This practice was also applied in the actual study.

SETTING

Monrovia the capital city of the Republic of Liberia was the physical location of this study. Monrovia is 35.52 km² with a population of over one million people. Monrovia is one of the poorest cities in West Africa. The city is built on Cape Mesurado along the Atlantic Coast in Montserrado County, Liberia (LISGIS, 2014). The city was hardest hit by the 2014 EVD outbreak recording more than 60% of all EVD cases and mortality in the country (WHO, 2015). Most Liberians depend on the city for trade and jobs, thereby causing a fluid population movement across the country which may have exposed the city to the high rate of EVD mortality. EVD which is known to be among the most virulent pathogens that infect humans and non-human primates poses a great danger to poor resource countries such as Liberia. The Liberian government was not and is currently not equipped to contain and treat EVD. Panic and fear would grip every household or the entire community when an individual is seen showing signs of EVD. Early symptoms of EVD include fever, headache, body aches, cough, stomach pain, vomiting, and diarrhea and death within days (Leroy, Gonzalez & Baize, 2011).

In Monrovia and Liberia as a whole the concept of virus or disease and illness in general, is frequently associated with the world of spirits (gods).

These spirits which they believed to be either 'good' or 'bad' impact human lives in both good and bad ways (Hewlett & Amola, 2003). Almost everyone including the research participants I met and greeted in Monrovia and asked how they were doing would answer saying "by his grace I am alive." They believe that their only reason for surviving EVD was their gods because hospitals and health workers had no answers to their plight. The word "grace" was commonly mentioned by all participants during the pilot testing thus giving the researcher cause for using it as the interview code to replace participants' names. Thus the research interview records identified all participants as "GRACE" followed by a couple of assigned numbers.

The recruitment process began after obtaining IRB approval. In the first week, letters of invitation to participate in the study (see Appendix D) were distributed to all research partners. In the same week, I began to make phone calls and home visits to potential participants explaining to them the reason for the study. Some of the potential participants responded favorably to the first approach and voluntarily agreed to participate in the study, while others were initially hesitant but later agreed to participate. By the second week, flyers bearing the researcher's contact information were conspicuously posted in strategic areas in the communities inviting EVD survivors and their family caregivers to participate in the study. The flyers paid off well by yielding favorable responses.

By the 10th day into the recruitment process, 6 EVD survivors along with their respective family caregivers (6 family caregivers) had agreed to participate in the study. By the 15th day of the recruitment process, an additional 4 EVD survivors and their respective family caregivers (4 family caregivers) also agreed to participate in the study. This amounted to 10 EVD survivors and 10 family caregivers as proposed for this study. The remaining 10 participants were recruited in the first and second weeks respectively as follows; 2 from MOH & SW, 2 from LNRC, and 2 from MSF. Additionally, 2 academicians and 2 members of the media were also recruited to participate in the study. The recruitment process was concluded with 30 participants and subsequently followed by the interview process. The entire recruitment process was in line with the researcher's time and schedule.

DEMOGRAPHICS

As mentioned earlier, a total of 30 voluntary adult participants were recruited and participated in the research study including 10 EVD survivors, 10 family caregivers, and 10 additional participants that included government officials, NGO staff, academicians, and reporters from the media. These latter 10 participants were 2 officials of government from the Ministry of Health and Social Welfare, 2 health workers from Médecins Sans Frontier, 2 health workers from the Liberia National Red Cross, 2 academicians from the communities, and 2 members of the media who covered the 2014 EVD outbreak. The names of the voluntary study participants remained confidential; no first or last names appeared on observation, interview, or researcher notes. The audio or tape recordings contained no identifying information to include first or last names. For the purpose of recordkeeping, a designated code was used to identify each of the participants (see Table 1).

TABLE 1
STUDY PARTICIPANTS

Participants' code	Organization	Location	Gender
GRACE M01GO	Ministry of Health	IOO	M
GRACE M02GO	Ministry of Health	IOO	M
GRACE F03NG	Liberia National Red Cross	IOCR	F
GRACE M04NG	Liberia National Red Cross	IOCR	M
GRACE F29NG	Médecins Sans Frontier	IOCR	F
GRACE F30NG	Médecins Sans Frontier	IOCR	F
GRACE MOFAC	Academician	IO	M
GRACE M28AC	Academician	IO	M
GRACE M09ME	Media	IO '	M
GRACE F27ME	Media	IO	F
GRACE F6SUV	EVD Survivor	IOHCRCC	F
GRACE F7SUV	EVD Survivor	IOHCRCC	F
GRACE M8SUV	EVD Survivor	IOHCRCC	M

GRACE M10SUV	EVD Survivor	IOHCRCC	M
GRACE F11SUV	EVD Survivor	IOHCRCC	F
GRACE F12SUV	EVD Survivor	IOHCRCC	F
GRACE M13SUV	EVD Survivor	IOHCRCC	M
GRACE F14SUV	EVD Survivor	IOHCRCC	F
GRACE M15SUV	EVD Survivor	IOHCRCC	M
GRACE M16SUV	EVD Survivor	IOHCRCC	M
GRACE F17FCG	Family Caregiver	IOHCRCC	F
GRACE F18FCG	Family Caregiver	IOHCRCC	F
GRACE F19FCG	Family Caregiver	IOHCRCC	F
GRACE M20FCG	Family Caregiver	IOHCRCC	M
GRACE F21FCG	Family Caregiver	IOHCRCC	F
GRACE M22FCG	Family Caregiver	IOHCRCC	F
GRACE F23FCG	Family Caregiver	IOHCRCC	F
GRACE M24FCG	Family Caregiver	IOHCRCC	M
GRACE M25FCG	Family Caregiver	IOHCRCC	M
GRACE F26 FCG	Family Caregiver	IOHCRCC	F

Note. Codes used to protect participants' privacy.

"GRACE" participant's code name, "M" participant's gender (Male), "F" participant's gender (Female), "01, 03, 07"... assigned numbers, "GO" government official. "NG" nongovernmental organization, "AC" academician, "ME" media, "SUV" EVD survivor, "FCG" family caregiver. In the location column, "I" interview, "O" observation, "O" office where the interviews and observations were conducted. "CR" conference room where the interview and observation was conducted. "H" participant's home where the interviews and observations were conducted and "CC" community center where the interviews and observations were conducted. The 10 EVD survivors and their 10 family caregivers are previous and current residents of the selected communities and they directly experience the impact of EVD. Therefore, their input supported the study to achieve its goal. The other 10 participants mentioned above were recruited to support the study achieve data saturation. These additional participants were individuals who provided care and other services for EVD patients during the 2014 EVD outbreak.

DATA COLLECTION

After obtaining IRB approval from Walden University (number: 10-04-16-0166341), formal letters of invitation to participate in the study were given to the three research partners at MOH & SW, MSF, and LNRC. Subsequently, separate meetings were held with the Director at LERT at the MOH & SW, the Head of Mission at MSF, and the Director at the LNRC respectively. The purpose of the research was explained during the meetings including the procedures for participant selection. Permission was granted when the researcher asked to use their respective conference room for interviews and or observations. The research partners agreed to participate in the study. An Informed Consent Form was given to each partner at the meeting that explained the purpose and nature of the study, the time commitment involved, the rights of the participants, and the possible risks associated with the study. The three partners returned the Informed Consent Form agreeing to participate in the Study. Another meeting was scheduled in the same manner to meet with other staff to request their participation in the study. At this meeting, three more participants each from MOH & SW, MSF, and LNRC read, understood, and signed the Informed Consent Form to participate in the study. These amounted to a total of six participants from the research partners.

Also during these meetings with the research partners, names and contact information of EVD survivors and their family caregivers was received from the partners. The researcher then proceeded by contacting the EVD survivors and their family caregivers by phone and home visits. During the phone calls and home visits, the researcher first introduced himself and explained the purpose of the research. Some of the participants were very enthusiastic from the first approach while some were hesitant from the beginning. After making follow-up calls and visits, these unwilling participants became excited to participate in the study. Letters of invitation were given to the participants, and each replied favorably. A meeting with the EVD survivors and their family caregivers was scheduled at the conference room of the LNRC. A total of 20 participants (10 EVD survivors and 10 family caregivers attended the meeting). During the meeting, each participant received an Informed Consent Form that explained the purpose and nature of the study, the time commitment, the rights of the participants, and the possible risks associated with the study. For the sake of those that could not read; the researcher then read and explained in detail, and the participants confirmed their understanding of the research purpose and all the conditions associated with the study. All 20 participants signed and returned the Informed Consent Forms.

Posters bearing the researcher's contact information were conspicuously posted in the communities inviting individuals such as academicians and members from the media to participate in the study. In this vein, two academicians and two members of the media contacted the researcher expressing their willingness to participate in the study. Formal letters of invitation to participate in the study were extended to the four additional participants. A meeting was scheduled, and during the meeting, each participant received an Informed Consent Form that explained the purpose and nature of the study, the time commitment involved, the rights of the participants, and the possible risks associated with the study. The four participants read, understood, signed and returned the Informed Consent Forms. This made an overall total of 30 participants who read, understood, and signed the Informed Consent Forms to participate in the study. Interviews with participants were scheduled on a one-to-one basis.

INTERVIEW PROTOCOL

All the interviews began by providing and reading the script on the Qualitative Interview Protocol (see Appendix A). At that time, the researcher shared detailed information about the study, including the social implications of the study and the next steps in the research process. The data collection process included the use of field notes, an audio tape recorder, and a notebook or laptop computer. An audiotape recorded each session and later transcribed into written form for analysis. The information was coded and segmented to allow for easy analysis of the coded data using the NVivo software program. Generally, each participant was asked to give their meaning or perception about Ebola. The interview process then continued with the semi-structured interview questions, allowing the participant to elaborate and to ask follow-up questions as necessary. Walden University approved open-ended interview questions were used for this study. All EVD survivors and family caregivers answered the same questions. While the research partners including government officials, NGO staff, academicians and members of the media all answered the same questions (see Appendix A). Through follow-up questions, the researcher clarified some stated points and sought more meanings into a particular theme of the study. This way, the researcher easily analyzed and compared themes from participants' perceptions.

Interviews of the 10 EVD survivors and their 10 family caregivers were conducted in their respective homes and with consent of the participants. The remaining 10 interviews were conducted in the conference rooms of MSF and LNRC, and community centers, and interviews of government officials, NGO staff, academicians and members of the media were conducted in their respective offices and conference rooms. With the consent of participants, the researcher tape-recorded all the interviews. During each interview, a notebook was used to take notes and to make reflections to responses. Before each interview, participants were told that they can stop the interview at any time once they feel uncomfortable to continue the process. At their request, participants received copy of the interview script. The goal of the interviews was: (a) to obtain understanding of the experiences of research participants as it relates to EVD; (b) to understand the social, economic, and policy factors that contributed to the spread of EVD; (c) to understand how residents of Monrovia coped with the threat of EVD and its impact or social stigma on survivors, family caregivers and the public in general; and (d) to understand if the Liberian government's mandatory cremation policies and the banning of public gatherings further exacerbated the spread of EVD.

Each face-to-face in-depth interview lasted approximately 45 minutes to one hour as originally planned by the researcher. Data collection also included diary accounts of some participants of their experience with EVD. The researcher collected the diaries of participants during the data collection process and returned them at the end of the data collection process. The information in these diaries helped the researcher understand the participants' experiences and perceptions about EVD. The researcher asked follow-up questions as needed while maintaining focus on the central themes. The data collected were coded and analyzed and applied specific codes to selected quotations and noted the frequency of the major themes. Each participant had a 10-15 minute debriefing session to reflect on the interview process and questions that may not have been covered adequately during the interview. The participant also clarified any doubts about the interview at that point. No variations from the data collection plan, as previously presented within Chapter 3, or unusual circumstances in data collection occurred. At the end of each interview, the participant was thanked for their participation and informed that she or he may be called upon again if necessary for follow-up interviews. Each participant was initially assured of the confidentiality of their information and participation.

OBSERVATION PROTOCOL

In addition to information gathered during interviews, participants were also observed. Each meeting or interview time varied between 45 minutes to one hour. During observation, an observation data collection form (see Appendix C) was used to record field notes and research reflections. The researcher spent time observing participants during interviews or meetings. This involved observing and taking notes to describe activities, interactions, reactions, and discourses relating to the impact of EVD on participants. Hand-written notes were taken during and after data collection and throughout data analysis, and created a field log. The field log consisted of the researcher's notes during the interviews and observations. These notes were reviewed many times to ensure that the researcher had fairly represented the participants' responses and to reduce any biases in the research findings. All interview data, and the researcher's notes were saved on a hard drive protected password and a locked cabinet to which only the researcher have access.

This case study observation required that the researcher follow the activities of those being explored through interactions. The researcher captured in field notes a detailed description of activities relating to participants' activities or behaviors. The behavior of each participant was explained and interpreted. The researcher was principally observing activities and interactions, but questions were also asked for the purpose of clarification and individual participants were asked about their experiences, seeking to bring to light logics, concerns, and meanings that emerge from the observational activities. Discussions and interviews were recorded manually in field notes, to provide more detailed information. The researcher digitally recorded informal interviews or discussions for later transcription.

On the observational data collection template, the researcher noted re-cordkeeping information such as the date, the beginning time, the ending time, site, and the study participant code/label. Additional note taking areas, on the template, included descriptive notes referencing physical setting, sequential activities/actions, and non-verbal/body behavior. Areas for noting interactions with other persons during general meetings were available. The template further included an area for the researcher additionally observed items; the area was also used for the researcher's notes post observation.

DATA ANALYSIS

The purpose of data analysis according to Polit and Beck (2012) is to organize, provide structure to and elicit actual meaning from narrative data. This process is a data reduction and sense-making effort that takes the qualitative material and attempts to identify core consistencies and meanings therein (Patton, 2001). Qualitative data analysis is an analytical process designed to condense raw data into categories or themes based on valid inferences. This process relied on in-ductive reasoning and entailed the researcher to create generalizations from specific observations. Data analysis is an important part of qualitative research process because it allows the researcher to fit data together, make the invisible obvious, and draw general conclusions about the phenomenon (Polit and Beck, 2012). Qualitative data analysis is an analytical process designed to condense raw data into categories or themes based on valid inferences.

Data analysis for this qualitative study was based on configuring collected data into understandable information (Merriam, 2009). The data analysis pro-cess occurred throughout the duration of this study. This study employed the use of NVivo 10 to manage, organize, and keep track of data. These included raw data such as interviews, questionnaires, observations, and audio recordings.

DATA ANALYSIS PLAN

Before data analyses, the researcher listed each of the research questions along with various interview questions to show alignment. The reason for this was so that the data analysis plan to guide the data analysis process aimed at en-suring that interviews aligned with the research questions and data presented sequentially. Having received training on qualitative data analysis using NVivo software design, the researcher used the software to group information collected into themes and codes accordingly. For example, during the interviews process, all participants used words or group of words such as "fear", "by the grace of god", "denial", "neglect", "poor facility", "burial rites", no medicine" among others. In using this tool, the researcher attempted to answer the research questions identified in Chapter 1 by analyzing interview questions based on themes also identified in Chapter 2. The case study data analysis framework of Bandura (1997) was used because at its core is description of things as they appear in peoples' lived experiences. The process of reducing data into meaning units begins with immersing in and dwelling with the data and repeatedly reading the transcripts, alongside the field notes and recalling the observations and occurrences recorded during the interviews (Merriam, 2009).

This process helped the researcher to identify and extract significant statements from the data. The researcher applied two steps to accomplish this goal: Step 1: using NVivo 10 software, interview data were transcribed and categorized by establishing codes. The researcher ensured that the interview transcripts were read through and recordings listened to thus creating the opportunity to make marginal notes. This process supported the theory of using the line-by-line coding according to Yin (2014) recommendations for qualitative research. In this regard, this study followed the exact procedures when analyzing the observation field notes and reflections. NVivo 10 ensured a content analysis process for all documents. Step 2: NVivo 10 software was used to initiate themes or patterns. Accordingly, the themes and disparities that transpired from the coded and categorized data determined the key findings. These were analyzed in accordance to the central and related research questions for the study and interpreted according to the theoretical framework and the literature review. To the best of the researcher's knowledge, no discrepant cases emerged through the data analysis.

EVIDENCE OF TRUSTWORTHINESS

Standards of quality in research emphasize concepts of objectivity, validity, reliability, rigor, and honesty through reporting of research results. The standards of trustworthiness and quality for this study were emphasized on the concepts of credibility, validity, transferability, dependability, and confirmability through the reporting of research findings (Lincoln & Guba, 1985). This process entailed checking, confirming, making sure, and being confident that the researcher incrementally ensured reliability and validity and consequently rigor of the study. During this research process, the researcher incorporated validity and verification strategies. These included pre-testing the interview questions, and ensuring that the study's instrument was valid and measured what it was supposed to measure to attain reliability and validity. Research quality is when the research work conforms to the methodology of the study (Yin, 2014).

To ensure trustworthiness, Lincoln and Guba (1985) argued that the researcher must demonstrate that transition from raw data to informed data is valid. Trustworthiness can be achieved in a study when there is confidence in the truth (credibility) of the findings, and that the findings should have applicability (transferability) in other contexts. Trustworthiness ensures the findings are consistent (dependability) and could be repeated, and can demonstrate a degree of neutrality (confirmability) in a manner in which the results of the study were shaped by the respondents and not researcher bias, motivation, or interest (Lincoln & Guba, 1985). Each of the voluntary research participants experienced the impact of EVD, and they were very articulate in their responses during the observations and interviews process.

CREDIBILITY

Credibility refers to the confidence participants have in the truthfulness of the findings of a particular study (Polit & Beck, 2012). Merriam (2009) agreed that qualitative research study is considered credible when it portrays an accurate description of the human experience that people who also share the same experience would immediately recognize and find it believable. For this study, credibility was established through prolonged engagement with research participants which included the incorporation of method and data triangulation.

Prolonged engagement according to Polit and Beck (2012) is the investment of sufficient time collecting data to develop an in-depth understanding of the phenomenon. This process of prolonged engagement enabled the researcher to test for misinformation and distortions and to ensure saturation of relevant categories. In addition to being able to gather in-depth information, the prolonged engagement of research participants also resulted in building rapport and trust. The researcher spent sufficient time with each EVD survivor, family caregiver, government officials, NGO staff, academicians, and members of the media so that useful, accurate and rich data could be obtained to understand the phenomenon better. The prolonged engagement was fortified with some follow-ups interviews. The researcher followed the strategy of studying the phenomenon using multiple data sources. The triangulation of the analyzed data created ranges in personal perspectives regarding the conceptions intrinsic to the theoretical and conceptual framework of the study. Triangulation refers to the use of multiple reference points to draw conclusions about what constitutes truth (Polit & Beck, 2012) aimed at capturing a more complete and contextualized portrait of the phenomenon. Triangulation for this study was achieved by engaging in both methods and data triangulation:

- Method triangulation was achieved by using both the initial in-depth case study interviews and follow-up interviews which are two different data collection methods (Merriam, 2009). These two approaches ensured data collection from two different viewpoints and prevented biases and deficiencies usually associated with using single data collection method; the preliminary literature review helped the researcher to set the entire interview process.
- Data triangulation was achieved through an extensive review of relevant literature during the study. Furthermore, data triangulation was attained by collecting data from EVD survivors, family caregivers, government officials, NGO staff, academicians, and members of the media. These six different perspectives facilitated the researcher to gain a complete understanding of participants lived experiences as they described them (Merriam, 2009).

The researcher training in advanced qualitative courses at Walden University also contributed to the credibility of this study. The importance of the researcher experience is based on the fact that the researcher is the main instrument in qualitative study; as such the experience of a qualitative researcher contributes substantially to the outcome of the study (Patton, 2001).

TRANSFERABILITY

Transferability is the second criterion for establishing trustworthiness in qualitative research. According to Yin (2014), transferability refers to the degree to which the findings of a study can be applied to other contexts. Transferability entails the extent to which findings of a study may be generalized to other settings or groups (Polit & Beck, 2012). Streubert and Carpenter (2011) also consider transferability as referring to the probability that the findings have meanings to other in similar situations. The researcher during this study was acutely aware that the expectation of determining whether the findings fit or are transferable; rests with potential users. The researcher complied with Lincoln and Guba's (1985) criteria of providing the basis for making transferability judgment possible for potential users. Plans for transferability were enhanced by careful selection of participants and by providing sufficient descriptive data in the final report so that the consumers of the study may ably evaluate the applicability of findings to other circumstances.

The researcher ensured careful selection of participants by using only the approved sample criteria to select the best possible sample. The researcher utilized the Snowball sampling criteria to select participants for this study. Snowball sampling according to Patton (2001) is using one or two members of a group to identify persons who are typical of the phenomenon being studied. This study used the rich thick description recommended by Merriam (2009) to improve the transferability of this qualitative study. This strategy presented the setting and findings of the study and helped to implement the maximum variation of the typical sample. Additionally, the rich thick strategy also presented the participants, the data analysis procedures, and the findings. A rich thick strategy provides sufficient description to conceptualize the study. In this regard, the typicality of the sample for EVD survivors and family caregivers in the communities this study selected was typical of the many communities that were hit by the EVD outbreak in Monrovia.

DEPENDABILITY

The third criterion for establishing trustworthiness in qualitative research is dependability which means data stability over time and conditions (Polit & Beck, 2012). Merriam (2009) referred to dependability in qualitative research as reliability or consistency to the extent that research findings can be generalized. In this direction, Merriam (2009) suggested that the strategies of triangulation, peer-review, reflexivity, and an audit trail can improve the dependability of a qualitative study. An audit trail, in this case study, presented a detailed account of the methods, procedures, and decisions for the study.

The researcher assured dependability of the study findings by ensuring that all processes of this research were consistent with the philosophical and methodological principles of a case study research (Merriam, 2009). The researcher ensured that methods of data collection, analysis, including interpretation were explained clearly for others to verify (Lincoln & Guba, 1985). The first requirement of methodological consistency was boosted when the researcher acquainted himself with the general principles of qualitative methodology and case study method before conducting this study. The second strategy was to overcome inconsistencies in the research process by describing in detail the various steps of data collection, analysis, and interpretation.

CONFIRMABILITY

The fourth criterion for trustworthiness, confirmability refers to objectivity or neutrality of the research data. In qualitative research, the perception of confirmability correlates with the idea of objectivity. According to Polit and Beck (2012), objectivity refers to the potential for congruence between two or more independent people that data's accuracy, relevance, and meaning. A closely related concept of neutrality as noted by Lincoln and Guba (1985) is the criterion that the reader can use to ascertain the degree to which the findings of the study are determined by actual views of participants and not the researcher's imagination. Consistent with Polit and Beck's (2012) position, the researcher was conscious that the findings had to reflect participants' true voice and conditions and not the researcher's uninformed biases and views. The researcher demonstrated full objectivity through reflexivity.

Reflexivity, as defined by Merriam (2009), is the way to reflect critically on oneself as a researcher. During qualitative research, potential bias must be realized immediately and corrected to enable the researcher to present an honest report thus avoiding subjectivity. This study was designed to maintain a log in which the personal beliefs and assumptions of the researcher were documented for the purpose of clarifications and reflections. Subjectivity and bias were minimized by applying strict protocols during data collection and analysis. Decisions made in this study were as objective as possible and that all findings were addressed through reflective commentary according to the log being maintained.

The researcher was conscious of the role his pre-understanding about EVD would have on the findings. In remedy, the researcher remained open to mechanisms that would enhance the self-reflective stance required to enter the research with an open mindset (Streubert & Carpenter, 2011). This openness was achieved through the process of reflexivity. The researcher provided findings that met the goal of the study, not the result of the biases and subjectivity of the researcher (Merriam, 2009). This study used the strategy of triangulation to improve the objectivity of the research. The triangulation strategy was done by constantly cross-checking data sources during analysis of the data. The researcher also made sure that the data collected and analyzed represented the experiences, views, and beliefs of the participants, and not the researcher.

RESULTS

Research participants for this study were divided into two interview groups namely: group 1 comprised of government officials, NGO staff, academicians, and members of the media (research partners) whereas group 2 consisted of EVD survivors and family caregivers. The researcher imported individual interview transcripts into NVivo for data management during analysis. Once all 30 transcripts were imported into the software, the researcher assigned nodes for data analysis related to the research questions guiding this study.

The interview transcripts were then read to gain familiarity with the contents of the transcripts. The researcher re-read the transcripts to pull the information apart into units of meaning that were assigned to each node. These units of meaning, or codes, were grouped into categories and themes. The themes were organized according to the research questions, as detailed in this chapter. This process led to the creation of the following five themes: (1) Descriptive overview of coping with the threat of EVD, (2) Social-cultural beliefs, practices, and economic factors related to EVD, (3) Nature of EVD experience, (4) Reactions towards EVD outbreak, and (5) Surviving EVD. The themes were arranged and presented by the research questions to which they relate, with overarching themes and categories related to EVD.

Data Presentation With Literature Support

In this section, the synthesized interview data are presented in the form of themes and categories. The data are supported by evidence (verbatim quotes from participants) to enhance audit trail credibility. As stated earlier, the data analysis process resulted in the creation of five themes and 32 categories as shown in Table 2 where each theme with its categories and data display is illustrated. Data display in this section represents verbatim quotes, themes, and categories generated from the analysis of data.

TABLE 2

Summary of Themes and Categories

Theme 1: Descriptive Overview of Coping with the Threat of EVD

1.	Defining characteristics of EVD	
	(a) Fear, ostracism and stigmatization	GRACE M05AC; GRACE F6SUV
	(b) Annihilation of sufferers actualities and possibilities	GRACE F30NG; GRACE M05AC
	(c) Lingering nature of the traumatic experience	GRACE F6SUV; GRACE F17FCG
	(d) Psychosomatic manifestations	GRACE F12SUV; GRACE F19FCG
	(e) Inescapability of EVD experience	GRACE M8SUV; GRACE F29NG
2.	Response to traumatizing nature of EVD	
	(a) Seeking self-preservation and protection	GRACE F11SUV
	(b) Transcending victimhood and empowering self	GRACE F7SUV

Theme 2: Social-cultural beliefs, practices, and economic factors related to EVD

1.	Explanation models of causation of EVD	
	(a) EVD as supernatural occurrence	GRACE F26FCG; GRACE M15SUV
	(b) EVD as a natural occurring disease	GRACE M16SUV; GRACE F26FCG
2.	Beliefs and practices to remedy EVD	
	(a) Remedying EVD through natural means	GRACE F6SUV; GRACE M16SUV
	(b) Remedying EVD through supernatural means	GRACE F26FCG; GRACE F17FCG
	(c) Remedying EVD through both natural and supernatural means	GRACE M13SUV; GRACE M15SUV

Theme 3: Nature of EVD experience

1. Defining moments of EVD experience

    (a) Role of the caring other in defining moments   GRACE M24FCG; GRACE F30NG

    (b) Vacillations between hope and despair   GRACE M24FCG; GRACE F30NG

2. Positive outcome

    (a) Improved personal hygiene and protection practices   GRACE F12SUV; GRACE M22FCG .

    (b) Improved self-awareness and health seeking behavior   GRACE F26FCG; GRACE M04NG

    (c) Improved clinical care practices   GRACE M25FCG; GRACE M16SUV

3. Negative outcome

    (a) Abandonment of culturally cherished practices   GRACE M25FCG; GRACE M16SUV

    (b) Loss of related others   GRACE M15SUV; GRACE M14SUV

    (c) Abandonment and rejection of sufferers   GRACE F12SUV; GRACE F6SUV

    (d) Isolation and ostracism

    (e) Stigmatization, shame and embarrassment

Theme 4: Reactions towards EVD outbreak

1. Reaction before, during and after EVD outbreak

    (a) Government response to the epidemic   GRACE M10SUV; GRACE M17SUV

    (b) NGO response to the epidemic   GRACE M10SUV

    (c) Public reaction during EVD Outbreak   GRACE M17SUV

    (d) Public reaction before EVD Outbreak   GRACE M09ME; GRACE F03NG

    (e) Public reaction after EVD Outbreak   GRACE M09ME

2. Symbolism of public reaction

    (a) Ignorance, misconceptions and lack of knowledge   GRACE F03NG; GRACE F27ME

Theme 5: Surviving EVD

1. The experience of surviving EVD

    (a) Physical implications of surviving   GRACE F27ME; GRACE M28AC

    (b) Psychological implications of surviving   GRACE M05AC; GRACE M13SUV

    (c) Social implications of surviving EVD   GRACE M01GO; GRACE F11SUV

    (d) Spiritual implications of surviving EVD   GRACE F29NG; GRACE F12SUV

    (e) Economic implications of surviving   GRACE M16SUV; GRACE M8SUV

Note: Themes and categories developed from data analysis EVD = Ebola virus disease.

TABLE 3

Theme 1: Descriptive Overview of Coping With the Threat of Ebola Virus Disease

---

Summary

1. Defining characteristics of coping with the threat of EVD
    - (a) Fear, ostracism and stigmatization (Data Display: GRACE M05AC; GRACE F6SUV)
    - (b) Annihilation of sufferers actualities and possibilities (Data Display: GRACE F30NG; GRACE M05AC)
    - (c) Lingering nature of the traumatic experience (Data Display: GRACE F6SUV; GRACE F17FCG)
    - (d) Psychosomatic manifestations (Data Display: GRACE F12SUV; GRACE F19FCG)
    - (e) Inescapability of EVD experience (Data Display: GRACE M8SUV; GRACE F29NG)
2. Response to traumatizing nature of EVD
    - (a) Seeking self-preservation and protection (Data Display: GRACE F7SUV)
    - (b) Transcending victimhood and empowering self (Data Display: GRACE M02GO)

Note: Theme and categories developed from data analysis. EVD = Ebola virus disease.

DEFINING CHARACTERISTICS OF COPING WITH THE THREAT OF EBOLA VIRUS DISEASE

EVD was experienced as a traumatic event that caused death and elicited fear and anxiety in all survivors, caregivers, and the general public. WHO (2014) considers a situation traumatic when there is a direct personal experience of an epidemic or event that involves actual or threatened death or serious injury. Trauma also includes a threat to one's physical integrity or witnessing an event that involves death, injury, or a threat to the physical integrity of another person. One participant described EVD trauma as intense fear, helplessness, and horror (GRACE F23FCG). Participants reported engaging in activities to reduce the painful anticipation experience and avoided further exposure to EVD. Such self-preservation and protection actions which enhance affected individuals' adaptive outcomes in the face of adversity. EVD infection was experienced by participants dependent on how the event affected their lives;

including circumstances that led them to consider it as positive or negative experience. Regardless of whether they classified their experience as positive or negative, EVD was experienced as "grave" and "life-threatening." The disease did not only affect participants' physical wellbeing, but it threatened their personhood. The features that made EVD traumatizing to participants relate to it causing fear, ostracism, and stigma. EVD annihilated sufferers' actualities and possibilities; lingering negative experience, psychosomatic manifestations and the fact that nearly everyone could get infected (inescapability).

FEAR, OSTRACISM, AND STIGMATIZATION

From the initial EVD outbreak, the threat of EVD was characterized by fear and panic. The concept of fear in a situation such as epidemic is defined by WHO (2014) to be an emotion caused by the belief that something is dangerous and has the potential to cause pain and threat. People in Monrovia, West Africa, and other parts of the world were subjected to fear as EVD ravaged their communities. A participant (academician) stated that "fear is an unpleasant emotion caused by the threat of danger, pain or harm while panic; a closely related state is a sudden uncontrollable fear or anxiety often causing wildly unthinkable behavior" (Data Display: GRACE M05AC). The findings show that the fear of infection resulted in widespread panic and hysteria (Data Display: GRACE F27ME). All participants stated that as the EVD outbreak was announced, fear and panic gripped nearly everyone.

People began to fear each other by avoiding one another. Everyone avoided getting close to one another for fear of getting infected. Individuals became suspicious about each other (Data Display: GRACE M02GO). "As for us who had the illness at home or in an isolation center, the fear toward us was so overwhelming that people would openly isolate and shun us" (Data Display: GRACE M10SUV). The findings also show that survivors and caregivers and the general public became suspicious of each other (Data Display: GRACE M05AC). As this continued, patients, survivors, caregivers, including health workers experienced ostracism and outright rejection as illustrated in Data Display: GRACE M05AC which contains statements related to fear, ostracism, and stigmatization.

ANNIHILATION OF SUFFERERS' ACTUALITIES AND POSSIBILITIES

Being infected with EVD posed a serious threat to the life of the sufferer even in the presence of health workers. Often sufferers became defenseless and were exposed to death (GRACE M28AC). The vulnerability of the sufferer even in the face of health care is apparent largely because of the dread experienced by the workers themselves. EVD interfered with their physical wellbeing, manifested in physical symptoms and the feeling of vulnerability led to a sense of despair and helplessness (GRACE F30NG).

- "We were told that whoever gets Ebola has no chances of survival. This news frightened us and was afraid the whole family would die because most people were sick. All we could do was to look up to God because health workers themselves were dying" (Data Display: GRACE M8SUV).
- "The fear and dread of EVD were so much because it killed many within a short time, including wiping out entire families" (Data Display: GRACE M02GO).
- "The EVD experience made me think that if ever the disease were to break out again, I would rather kill myself early enough before I get infected to avoid the intense suffering, pain, vomiting, and diarrhea" (Data Display: GRACE F17FCG)

The feeling of helplessness and desperation was greater when health workers became unwilling to help EVD patients; they too were afraid of being infected (Data Display: GRACE F18FCG). Survivors received news of their diagnosis with intense feelings of terror, fear, and anxiety, far beyond the danger usually associated with another epidemic. Caregivers experienced the anticipation of the onset of symptoms and their death as a time of worry and despair about the future. This despair appeared to have been exacerbated by witnessing the excruciating pain and suffering of their patients (GRACE M04NG).

LINGERING NATURE OF THE TRAUMATIC EXPERIENCE

Participants reported that they experienced the trauma of EVD for prolonged periods, lingering on, even after declaring the end of the epidemic (GRACE F6SUV; GRACE F17FCG).

- "When I recently heard that another EVD outbreak happened in Paynesville, fear gripped me. I felt pity for the affected individuals. I prayed to God that they also survive like I did. When I saw them on television, I recalled my experience in the isolation ward. I felt their suffering" (Data Display: GRACE M10SUV).
- "When I reflect on this whole EVD experience, I feel a lot of agony and pain in my heart. I sometimes feel angry because my life has changed since I became an EVD survivor. I feel very lonely these days" (Data Display: GRACE F6SUV).

The persistence of the traumatic experience was witnessed again when another EVD outbreak occurred in a neighboring community. The situation made clear evidence that EVD triggers feeling of threat and anxiety leading to psychosomatic manifestations and symptoms such as fear, panic as well as sadness. Hewlett and Amola (2003) defined psychosomatic manifestation as a condition in which an individual's psychological stresses adversely affect their physiological (somatic) functioning, usually due to their aroused emotional state.

PSYCHOSOMATIC MANIFESTATIONS

Participants reported that their corporeal reactions were emotional, physical, mental or behavioral (Data Display: GRACE F12SUV; GRACE F19FCG). The term corporeal refers to the physical body and the physical symptoms participants experienced (Hewlett & Amola, 2003). The disease impacted them with anxiety, irritability, depression, anger, mood swing, physical symptoms like chronic aches and pain. They reported difficulty sleeping including nightmares. Participants also reported experiencing a plethora of strong emotional reactions such as sadness, anger, and anxiety as they anticipated or recovered from EVD (Data Display: GRACE F19FCG; GRACE F17FCG).

INESCAPABILITY OF THE TRAUMATIC EXPERIENCE

Participants experienced the traumatic experience of EVD either as they anticipated, experienced or witnessed the epidemic, regardless of whether they were survivors or caregivers or members of the general public. The severity of the infection alongside the scary clinical presentation created an impression that no one was safe. The following verbatim quotes support this category, which signify inescapability of EVD.

- "When my blood test results came and I was confirmed positive for Ebola disease, I was worried. I concluded right away that I wouldn't get heal as portrayed in the media and as the public was insinuating about the disease. I gave up and waited to die. At that point, I decided to be left alone until my death" (Data Display: GRACE M8SUV).
- "As the epidemic began to reach its height, more and more caregivers came in for treatment because they had started to experience signs and symptoms of EVD falsely. When we examined them, most of the times we found they were not ill in an actual sense. Everyone was confused, as a nurse for over 25 years, I too was confused" (Data Display: GRACE F29NG).
- "I was worried because a family member, who had already succumbed to Ebola after looking after another relative, had spent time with me in the same house. I have been involved in the care of all these people, we stayed in the same room and shared the same bed" (Data Display: GRACE F17FCG).

As highlighted in the verbatim quotes, survivors strongly believed that they would not survive the onslaught of EVD, especially in light of the media courage of the epidemic as well as considering the clinical picture of the disease. Caregivers too believed that they would become infected and die from EVD related complications, apparently bolster by scary stories in the media. Health workers panicky responses and behavior and their repeated exposure to the patients (Data Display: GRACE F29NG). This feeling of inevitability is congruent with Chan (2014) affirmation that EVD epidemics are characterized by media hype and mostly sensationalist accounts making them to be widely recognized and feared.

While survivors anticipated their death and caregivers expected to contract EVD, all participants responded to the illness in ways that may be categorized as struggling to secure or protect their survival or wellbeing, which is akin to the concept of resilience. Helman, (2007) defined resilience as a psychological process developed in response to intense life stressors that facilitates healthy functioning. The notion of resilience should be understood as survivors', caregivers' and community's ability to maintain relatively stable lives despite the various challenges and threats through specific interventional steps.

RESPONSE TO TRAUMATIZING NATURE OF EBOLA VIRUS DISEASE

- People reacted with anxiety because EVD is a killer disease which spreads rapidly over a short period. Affected persons were shunned because by touching the body fluids of the person with EVD, it was easy to get infected too. In general, people reacted frantically due to danger of the disease (Data Display: GRACE M05AC).
- "Neighbors and relatives shunned and avoided us because of fear of infection. People believed that if they visited me, they would most likely contract EVD" (Data Display: GRACE F6SUV).
- "They feared death because they knew anyone who got infected would die. The deaths of health workers even made the situation worse because they believed health workers are skilled and knowledgeable on health issues" (Data Display: GRACE F03NG).
- "When the epidemic was declared as EVD, neighbors, friends, and relatives who knew that EVD was in our home became reluctant to visit us. For more than four months, people avoided us. Whenever people saw our family members or us, they feared us because of the misconception that whoever came to our family, left with an EVD infection. The shunning became common, even up to now some people are scared to visit us, they think that our home is unsafe" (Data Display: GRACE M8SUV).

Participants spoke frequently about ostracism and stigmatization. Hewlett and Amola (2003) defined ostracism as the act of ignoring and excluding an individual or group of individuals, and the related act of social rejection. Ostracism causes an individual to lose his or her self-esteem, self-control, meaningful existence and elicits psychological pain. As ostracism continued, more fear piled as patients, caregivers, and close family members were stigmatized. Stigma is an attribute or characteristic that is profoundly discrediting to the individual possessing the attribute or characteristic (Farmer, 2001). People or communities associated with any form of stigma such as EVD suffer from social rejection, violence, and diminished quality of life (De Roo et al., 1995). Participants reported incidences of being discredited and disadvantaged for being infected with EVD (GRACE F6SUV; GRACE F17FCG).

Participants also explained that the frightening disease pictures exacerbated by the media reports resulted in unprecedented levels of fear and panic which led to intense stigmatization (Data Display: GRACE F17FCG; GRACE F11SUV). Participants also stated that the EVD situation was so tense that many survivors and their caregivers were not allowed to return home from the hospital. Their clothes and properties were burned and some marriages dissipated needlessly (Data Display: GRACE M28AC; GRACE F27ME). Survivors' and caregivers' children were told not to touch them, and wives were ordered to go back to their parents' homes by husbands who were too afraid to take them back (Data Display: GRACE M28AC).

SEEKING SELF-PRESERVATION AND PROTECTION

The study found both survivors and caregivers responded resiliently by engaging in some actions and processes to protect and immunize themselves against the traumatizing effects of EVD infection. This involved exercising better caution and personal protection strategies as affirmed in the following verbatim quotes.

- "When I hear there was another EVD outbreak, I decided I would make cleanliness as a priority and become more careful. So I started cleaning my home with chlorine solution. I became more hygienic and avoided situations that could bring back the disease. I stopped shaking people's hands" (Data Display: GRACE F7SUV).
- "I was very careful when caring for patients especially the very sick ones during the 21 days so that I did not contract EVD. As I waited to see if I would develop any signs of EVD, I continue to do my work with patients. We went out for health education and counseling sessions to help calm the community. This helped to keep me calm and focused" (Data Display: GRACE F30NG).

TRANSCENDING VICTIMHOOD AND EMPOWERING SELF

The defining features of EVD experience were related to annihilation of survivors' and caregivers' actualities and possibilities; including the lingering nature of the traumatic experience, psychosomatic manifestations, and inescapability of the experience. Survivors and caregivers who had this experience responded by seeking opportunities for self-preservation by keeping away from situations that could aggravate their wellbeing. Also, survivors and caregivers said that they engaged in combative actions to protect themselves and others from such traumatic experience (Data Display: GRACE M02GO).

The concept of threat is explained by De Roo et al. (1995) as a person or a disease likely to cause damage or death. In 2014, the EVD outbreak was a major threat to the people of Liberia. Participants expressed both implicitly and explicitly that the threat and the experience of EVD infection were traumatizing and upsetting. De Roo et al. (1995) considers trauma as severe emotional shock and pain caused by an extremely upsetting experience. Giorgi (1997) argued that trauma as a very difficult or unpleasant experience can cause someone to have mental or emotional problems usually for a long time. These unpleasant experiences equate to anticipating, witnessing, getting infected, and surviving EVD as survivor and caregiver.

TABLE 4

Theme 2: Social-cultural beliefs, practices, and economic factors related to Ebola Virus Disease

---

Summary

1. Explanation models of causation of EVD
   - (a) EVD as supernatural occurrence (Data Display: GRACE F26FCG)
   - (b) EVD as a natural occurring disease (Data Display: GRACE M16SUV)
2. Beliefs and practices to remedy EVD
   - (a) Remedying EVD through natural means (Data Display: GRACE F6SUV)
   - (b) Remedying EVD through supernatural means (Data Display: GRACE F17FCG)
   - (c) Remedying EVD through both natural and supernatural means (Data Display: GRACE M15SUV)

Note: Theme and categories developed from data analysis

EXPLANATION MODELS OF CAUSATION OF EBOLA VIRUS DISEASE

The emergence of EVD resulted in several explanatory models to help health workers and the communities come to terms with what EVD was to deal with the epidemic. This section highlights different perspectives (models) including practices that were used to mitigate the outbreak. Beliefs should be understood as tenets held by people in Monrovia and practices as peoples' actions based on established beliefs and related customs (Chan 2014). The socio-cultural beliefs and practices related to EVD, therefore, imply the various beliefs and practices held by Monrovians following EVD, including the cultural models Monrovians adopted to explain the origin of the strange illness. The type of explanatory model an individual or the community holds is critical because it influences how they interpret health messages. And how they seek health care in the face of illness including the course of treatment they may choose to follow (Tosh & Sampathkumar, 2014). A cultural explanatory model of an illness (CEMI) is an individual's socially transmitted understanding and explanation for a particular illness. The CEMI includes an individual's ideas about signs, symptoms, cause, treatment, prevention, and prognosis about the illness (Hewlett & Hewlett, 2005).

EBOLA VIRUS DISEASE AS SUPERNATURAL OCCURRENCE

Participants believed the supernatural theory and blamed satanic or evil spirits for the epidemic. They believed that EVD was a punishment by deities, witchcraft or sorcery for the EVD outbreak (Data Display: GRACE F26FCG). Participants explained that the theory that equated EVD to satanic or evil spirits attack was particularly common in the early days of the epidemic when it resulted in mysterious deaths (Data Display: GRACE M25FCG). This observation is similar to Hewlett and Amola (2003) that most Africans believe in spirits as their guiding forces. These spirits which are believed to be either 'good' or 'bad' impact human lives in both good and bad ways. That is, the good spirits are believed to protect humans against harm, misfortune or disease; whereas the bad spirits would inflict disease, misfortune or suffering. Helman (2007) confirmed that these models hold that disease may result from an internal imbalance within the body or may arise from negative external influences related to actions of bad spirits, witches or deities.

- "We thought they had been attacked by "Jinna" a form of supernatural beings or evil entity. It was widely believed the affected families were targeted by someone with evil powers who wanted to finish them off" (Data Display: GRACE M25FCG).
- "After the fever treatment had failed using the usual medications, we thought that the illness could have a spiritual aspect to it, may be the work of Satan" (Data Display: GRACE F19FCG).
- "Initially, my thoughts settled on the work of evil powers because of the circumstances under which the young babies died" (Data Display: GRACE F17FCG).

EBOLA VIRUS DISEASE AS NATURAL OCCURRING DISEASE

The findings show that in the initial stages of the EVD outbreak, most people believed that the mysterious illness was caused by "supernatural" forces. However, as the disease spread further, participants reported that many members of their community began to embrace the "natural" explanatory model, especially after confirmation of the outbreak. Despite confirming Ebola virus as the cause of the disease that spreads through contact from one person to another, some members of the community continued to hold EVD as a product of supernatural forces. While this opinion persisted, most people became convinced that EVD was a naturally occurring disease as stated in the following verbatim quotes.

- "Some of us thought it was severe malaria or diarrhea and others thought it was the usual nose bleeding that some people normally have" (Data Display: GRACE F6SUV).
- "For me, Ebola is a real disease although some people think it was a scam or magic. No one could explain the source of the scam or magic" (Data Display: GRACE M13SUV).
- "Some people said that Ebola came as a result of affected individuals eating monkeys. Others said that they ate infected pig" (Data Display: GRACE F18FCG).

BELIEFS AND PRACTICES TO REMEDY EBOLA VIRUS DISEASE

In the initial stages of the outbreak, people did not know what was causing these sudden and mysterious deaths of up to 26 people in one community in one week. Some individuals believed EVD was a common or regular disease that originated from infected wild animals contracted by humans by eating forbidden food or having contact with wild animals.

REMEDYING EBOLA VIRUS DISEASE THROUGH NATURAL MEANS

The practices participants reportedly used to deal with the EVD onslaught depended on whether they considered EVD a product of natural or supernatural occurrence. Those individuals who believed EVD was a common disease sought treatment from the regular clinics or hospitals.

- "I started to experience a headache, fever, vomiting and diarrhea. I immediately went for treatment to the clinic; my blood was tested. I went back home and took a dose of anti-malaria medication" (Data Display: GRACE F14SUV).Whereas, those who believed EVD had supernatural causes sought supernatural means to remedy the infection.
- "I initially started off with an ordinary fever, but in a couple of days, the fever became worse. I could not improve despite taking fever medication. So I decided to call a priest so that I could receive the sacraments for the sick before I went to a hospital. So when they gave me the sacraments, I was firm" (Data Display: GRACE M15SUV).The third group of community members unsure of how to categorize EVD opted for both natural and supernatural remedies as stated in the following verbatim quotes.
- "As prescribed by culture, when strange events such as illness strike people, some people go to small gods, deities for consultations; while others go for regular prayers for healing. As for me, I went for regular prayers and treatment. Several people prayed for me when I was still home before going to the hospital" (Data Display: GRACE M13SUV). As illustrated in the above verbatim quotes, some participants reported that early in the epidemic, they sought treatment from regular clinics and hospitals when they began to experience symptoms

of ill-health such as a headache, diarrhea, and fever. Others decided to seek supernatural remedies from established places of worship such as churches, mosques and healing places operated by locally revered prophets and prophetesses, and spiritualists and healers.

Table 5

Theme 3: Social-cultural Beliefs, Practices, and Economic Factors Related to Ebola Virus Disease

---

Summary

1. Defining moments of EVD experience (Data Display: GRACE M01GO; GRACE M09ME)
    (a) Role of the caring other in defining moments (Data Display: GRACE M24FCG; GRACE F30NG)
    (b) Vacillations between hope and despair (Data Display: GRACE F12SUV; GRACE M22FCG)
2. Positive outcome (Data Display: GRACE F26FCG; GRACE M04NG)
    (a) Improved personal hygiene and protection practices (Data Display: GRACE F26FCG; GRACE M04NG)
    (b) Improved self-awareness and health seeking behavior (Data Display: GRACE F30NG; GRACE M09ME; GRACE F29NG)
3. Negative outcome (Data Display: GRACE M25FCG; GRACE M16SUV)
    (a) Abandonment of culturally cherished practices (Data Display: GRACE M25FCG; GRACE M16SUV)
    (b) Loss of related others (Data Display: GRACE F23FCG; GRACE F17FCG)
    (c) Abandonment and rejection of sufferers (Data Display: GRACE M15SUV; GRACE M14SUV)
    (d) Isolation and ostracism (Data Display: GRACE F12SUV; GRACE F6SUV)
    (e) Stigmatization, shame and embarrassment (Data Display: GRACE M10SUV; GRACE M17SUV)

Note: Theme and categories developed from data analysis.

DEFINING MOMENTS OF EBOLA VIRUS DISEASE EXPERIENCE

In this section, the responses of participants during, before, and after EVD are explored. The Liberian government had in the past responded successfully to epidemics such as tuberculosis, cholera, and malaria by instituting some defined mechanisms that addressed the situation. The reason for these successes is based on the fact that they understood the etiology of these diseases supported by drugs that cured the diseases. EVD on the other hand, is a strange disease which currently has no cure and finding a defined mechanism has been a challenge. Health facilities in Monrovia are poorly equipped and medical staff lack training (Jerving, 2014).

The banning of public gathering and the mandatory cremation of EVD victims were designed by the Liberian government to stop the spread of EVD. However, these regulations were met with resentment among members of the communities. Participants reported that the policy to ban public gatherings further contributed to the spread of the disease because community members went into the streets to protest the ban (GRACE M24FCG; GRACE F30NG; GRACE M04NG). During the protest, some EVD patients ran away from the quarantining (isolation) centers. Some isolation centers were looted by protesters, thus exposing the communities to further disease contamination (GRACE M09ME).

ROLE OF THE CARING OTHER IN DEFINING MOMENTS

The rapid spread and high rate of mortality drew the attention of the international community operating in Liberia through the NGOs (GRACE M01GO). Participants reported that the NGOs attempted to address their needs as much as possible, but they too lack the resources necessary to contain the spread of EVD. The NGOs in collaboration with the government made every effort to contain the spread of the disease and to reduce mortality (GRACE M01GO; GRACE M09ME). These efforts were met with challenges as policy makers, and health care workers could not find a cure or defined mechanism to contain the disease (GRACE F27ME). The reaction of the public is described in light of the before, during, and the after declarations of the epidemic, followed by synthesis of the symbolism of public reaction to explain the reaction and behavior of the public.

VACILLATIONS BETWEEN HOPE AND DESPAIR

The findings show that EVD survivors and caregivers experienced simultaneous episodes of hoping for their desirable outcomes while at the same time anticipating the worst to happen. For survivors, their hope was hinged on surviving despite knowing that others had died (Data Display: GRACE F12SUV). Caregivers, on the other hand, hoped that despite their exposure to EVD, they would not seroconvert and get infected and eventually die from EVD (Data Display: GRACE F21FCG). The feeling of despair and hopelessness emerged from diverse reasons including the scary nature of EVD worsened by the media exaggeration. Hope was also lost because of the deplorable condition of health centers, poor social health education efforts, and heightened public awareness as highlighted in the following verbatim quotes.

- "Surviving from EVD was all I prayed for while in isolation ward. Although I wanted to survive, notwithstanding, I was not confident about my survival. I always used to reassure myself that the antibiotics and intravenous fluid I received might help me to recover" (Data Display: GRACE F12SUV).

- "When the government and health authorities finally declared the disease that was killing people was EVD, an overwhelming sense of despair and fear filled the entire city. My mind went back to several years ago to when the media used to report about Ebola in Uganda and the Congo. I concluded right away that my daughter who was in isolation would die because it was reported that no one can survive the disease. Since I was taking care of my daughter at home when she first started to show signs and symptoms of EVD, I knew that those who got affected were people who care for their sick relatives or friends" (Data Display: GRACE M22FCG).

POSITIVE OUTCOME

While the EVD experience was predominantly negative for most survivors and caregivers, participants reported that they also learned some positive lessons from their exposure to the outbreak. This positive growth led to improvements in personal hygiene and protection practices at homes and work places. Participants commonly agreed that the EVD outbreak helped them to gain self-awareness and health seeking patterns. In addition to these growth areas, survivors and caregivers who were health workers themselves reported that the experience made them to adopt better patient care practices during and in the aftermath of EVD.

IMPROVED PERSONAL HYGIENE AND PROTECTION PRACTICES

These findings appeared consistent with Usher and Grigg (2011) that state that the suffering and struggle to recover in the aftermath of a traumatic experience often yields remarkable transformation and positive growth. The act of cleanliness was perceived to keep the infection out of their homes and workplaces. In addition, participants also reported halting practices that could expose them to infection such as handshakes and sharing of personal effects as illustrated in the following verbatim quotes.

- "When I heard there was an EVD outbreak, my first reaction was fear. Later on, I calmed down. I decided that I would keep cleanliness as a priority and then become more careful and to stop sharing personal effects. So I started cleaning my home with chlorine. I became more conscious of dirt because I knew that it was dirt that would facilitate the entry of the disease to my home. I also focused on being more hygienic and avoided situations that could bring back the disease such as shaking people's hands" (Data Display: GRACE F26FCG).
- "The experience of being involved with EVD as a family caregiver has helped change my health behavior. These days I am more conscious about any disease. I do not take things for granted, be it a fever, diarrhea or vomiting. In any situation, I am a bit more conscious in my health practices now. Even in my clinical practice, this time when I am doing physical examinations, I put on exam gloves and regularly wash my hands with soap and water, which I never used to do before the outbreak" (Data Display: GRACE M04NG).

IMPROVED SELF-AWARENESS AND HEALTH SEEKING BEHAVIOR

These practices were consistent with health education programs carried out by NGOs and the Liberian health authorities. Participants further reported improvements in their self-awareness and health seeking behavior:

- "My practice as a nurse has changed a lot as a result of the EVD epidemic. I developed a greater self-awareness and my consciousness about infection became heightened" (Data Display: GRACE F30NG).

- "I created a particular column in my newspaper to educate the public how to practice good hygiene and to avoid contact with people. I ensured that the community radio stations played these Ebola-related messages educating the public to comply with the health team rules regarding safety measures to contain the spread of EVD" (Data Display: GRACE M09ME).

- "My practice as a midwife changed when I compare to what I used to do before the outbreak. Today, when I am with patients, I observe them very critically from head to toe. I now have quick plans, and I consult someone immediately if there is something I don't understand. I don't touch any patient when I go to perform delivery without the appropriate personal protective equipment" (Data Display: GRACE F29NG).

NEGATIVE OUTCOME

While EVD experience resulted in positive outcomes for some participants, nevertheless, the experience was negative for most survivors and caregivers. The negative experience relates to an abandonment of culturally cherished norms and traditional practices; the loss of loved ones; neglect and rejection of sufferers; stigmatization and shaming and embarrassment as well as isolation and ostracism. The section below highlights the negative outcomes experienced by participants.

- "When our loved ones died, we were not allowed to take part in the burial ceremony. We were not allowed to perform any traditional burial rites. Instead, our loved ones were interred by the epidemic response burial team. We were not to go closer to the burial sites or even say a prayer before the burial" (Data Display: GRACE M25FCG).

- "I was worried about dying and most importantly the fact that my fellow Christians would not pray for me at my burial" (Data Display: GRACE M16SUV).

ABANDONMENT OF CULTURALLY CHERISHED PRACTICES

As illustrated in the verbatim quotes above, the abandonment of the socio-cultural and religious burial practices bothered participants of which they dearly missed. While the abandonment of culturally or religiously sanctioned burial practices were believed to contain the spread of EVD, these practices were perceived commonly as negative by survivors and caregivers. These findings are consistent with results of studies conducted by De Roo et al. (1995) and Hewlett and Amola. (2003) indicating that the suffering experienced during the course and the aftermath of a traumatic experience yields several negative feelings and experiences. While these feelings were individualized, overall, it led to the generalization of these experienced as being negative. The study shows that the threat of EVD outbreaks ignited fear and heightened concern for wellbeing. It was characterized by avoidance of situations construed to compromise such wellbeing including established culture practices.

LOSS OF RELATED OTHERS

Another negative experience is the dramatic loss of lives, especially close relatives in a short span of time, which participants described as overwhelming and depressing. Caregivers reported that memories of their deceased relatives continued to affect them negatively leading to feelings of prolonged sadness and agony.

- "The feeling of losing many relatives in such a short span of time was incredibly overwhelming and depressing, coupled with the manner in which people feared us" (Data Display: GRACE F23FCG).
- "As my children and relatives died, neighbors wondered what the problem could be. The multiple and sudden deaths in my family were being discussed in the community. Our home became an ill omen as people marveled at us. People kept wondering why" (Data Display: GRACE F17FCG).

The loss of a loved one is often accompanied by a severe emotional burden sometimes resulting in major psychiatric complications of depression (Lazarus & Folkman, 1984). Evidence suggests that bereavement impacts individuals physically, cognitively, emotionally, interpersonally, behaviorally, and spiritually. The loss of a close relative may lead to an emotional reaction of fear, anger, guilt, confusion, sadness and loneliness (Helman, 2007).

ABANDONMENT AND REJECTION OF SUFFERERS

Another negative experience associated with EVD was the heightened desire by the public to stay healthy which resulted in survivors and caregivers being neglected and rejected by communities. The rejection of survivors and caregivers extended to family members and even by members of the health care team. As one participant stated; "when my diagnosis of EVD was confirmed, I felt neglected because not even the doctor or nurses wanted to handle my medical file. When I took the file to them, no one was there to receive it. When I was too weak to return to my bed from the bathroom, I slept on the floor. I became desperate. I thought of escaping from the hospital, but I could not do so because I was weak" (Data Display: GRACE M15SUV).

ISOLATION AND OSTRACISM

Participants reported that throughout the epidemic and thereafter, those who were known to have been connected to the illness were frequently isolated as highlighted in the verbatim quotes below.

- "I used to feel very bad when I realized the people I called my friends, with whom I grew up and went to school suddenly, would turn away and flee from me. Even some relatives advised their children to avoid my children and me" (Data Display: GRACE F12SUV).
- "When I was declared Ebola-free, and returned home from the isolation center, most people were not willing to stay with us. Schools in our community and nearby rejected my children and denied then entry because of my condition as an Ebola survivor" (Data Display: GRACE F6SUV).

When an individual or groups of individuals are intentionally ignored and excluded from society, they developed the feeling of ostracism (Hewlett and Amola, 2003). According to Hewlett and Amola (2003), their initial reactions to even the most minimal forms of ostracism are painful, distressing, and undesirable. When ostracized, individuals simultaneously experience social pain, distress, and their fundamental human needs of belonging, self-esteem, control, and their meaningful existence are threatened (De Roo et al., 1995).

STIGMATIZATION, SHAME, AND EMBARRASSMENT

The study findings show that survivors and caregivers were subjected to acts of prejudice and quarantine, and ultimately were ostracized by the other members of their communities. Because of these acts of rejection and isolation, survivors, caregivers, and their families were exposed to stigmatization, shame, and embarrassment. Stigma refers to socially devalued characteristics that expose a person to acts of prejudice and discrimination (De Roo et al., 1995). Participants reported that they were discriminated against, ridiculed by shop owners and shoppers, public transport operators, friends, acquaintances, neighbors, and family members.

Stigmatization occurs when a larger group of people expresses a negative attitude about socially unacceptable features of a smaller group. (Chan, 2014). This prejudicial association of the sufferer with the unwanted characteristic means the group is often blamed and embarrassed (Hewlett & Amola, 2003). Some participants reported that these prejudicial acts left them with the feelings of depression, sadness, and worry. Survivors reported that surviving EVD was met with extreme excitement and thankfulness, as the "impossible became a reality." The excitement derived from having conquered certain death from the dreaded illness. Survivors explained that their survival is credited to God Almighty and the health team members who played a significant role in their care and recovery (Data Display: GRACE M10SUV).

Other participants reported that the initial news of surviving EVD was received with disbelief (Data Display: GRACE M17SUV). Caregivers reported that caring for EVD patients and then being declared Ebola-free was an immensely pleasant experience. The experience was interpreted by caregivers as a sign of God listening to their ardent invocations and prayers. "So when we were declared Ebola-free, I thought that the time had not yet come for me to die like my relatives. I felt very blessed because, despite looking after several family members and initially taking part in their burial, I did not develop any sign of the disease. I was confident that God had listened to my prayers of preserving my life and our remaining family" (Data Display: GRACE M24FCG).

Table 6

Theme 4: Reactions towards Ebola Virus Disease Outbreak

Summary

1. Reaction before, during and after EVD outbreak
    (a) Government response to the epidemic (Data Display: GRACE M09ME).
    (b) NGO response to the epidemic (Data Display: GRACE F03NG).
    (c) Public reaction during EVD Outbreak (Data Display: GRACE F27ME; GRACE M28AC).
    (d) Public reaction before EVD Outbreak (Data Display: GRACE M05AC).
    (e) Public reaction after EVD Outbreak (Data Display: GRACE M05AC)
2. Symbolism of public reaction
    (a) Ignorance, misconceptions and lack of knowledge (Data Display: GRACE M01GO; GRACE F11SUV).

Note: Theme and categories developed from data analysis.

REACTION BEFORE, DURING AND AFTER EVD OUTBREAK

In this section, the responses of participants before and after EVD are explored. The Liberian government had in the past responded successfully to epidemics such as tuberculosis, cholera, and malaria by instituting some defined mechanisms that addressed the situation. The reasons for these successes are based on the fact that they understood the etiology of these diseases supported by drugs that cured the diseases. EVD is a strange disease which currently has no cure and finding a defined mechanism has been a challenge. Health facilities in Monrovia are poorly equipped and medical staff lack training (Jerving, 2014).

GOVERNMENT RESPONSE TO THE EPIDEMIC

The banning of public gathering and the mandatory cremation of EVD victims were designed by the Liberian government to stop the spread of EVD. However, these regulations were met with resentment among members of the communities. Participants reported that the policy to ban public gatherings further contributed to the spread of the disease because community members went into the streets to protest the ban (Data Display: GRACE M09ME).

NONGOVERNMENTAL ORGANIZATIONS RESPONSE TO THE EPIDEMIC

The rapid spread and high rate of mortality drew the attention of the international community operating in Liberia through the NGOs. Participants reported that the NGOs attempted to address their needs as much as possible, but they too lack the resources necessary to contain the spread of EVD. The NGOs in collaboration with the government made every effort to contain the spread of the disease and to reduce mortality. These efforts were met with challenges as policy makers, and health care workers could not find a cure or defined mechanism to contain the disease (Data Display; GRACE F03NG).

PUBLIC REACTION DURING EBOLA VIRUS DISEASE OUTBREAK

The Liberian government posed a ban on public gathering as means to contain the spread of EVD. Residents were not in any way given some incentives such as food and water to keep them in door. They had to go out daily to fetch food to survive. In this regard, the residents decided to ignore the ban to stay in door. They went into the streets to protest the ban (Data Display: GRACE F27ME). During the protest, some EVD patients ran away from the quarantining (isolation) centers. Some isolation centers were looted by protesters, thus exposing the communities to further disease contamination (Data Display: GRACE M28AC). The reaction of the public is described in light of the before, during, and the after declaration of the epidemic, followed by synthesis of the symbolism of public reaction to explain the reaction and behavior of the public toward EVD survivors and their family members.

PUBLIC REACTION BEFORE EBOLA VIRUS DISEASE OUTBREAK

The findings indicate that before the EVD outbreak, the surrounding communities in Monrovia were socially vibrant. Families and individuals carried on their routine businesses in their homes, shops, places of work and interacted freely with everyone. "I remember before Ebola, we had an excellent relationship with neighbors. We related well with each other. We would exchange visitations. The fact that my late mother was a well-known herbalist meant that she always had many visitors and patients who came to our home to pick up medicine for their sick children" (Data Display: GRACE M05AC). The verbatim quote above illustrates the existence of stable community where social interactions were "normal" before the outbreak and confirmation of EVD in Monrovia. Things were normal even during the early days of the outbreak, especially when the community had not yet fully conceptualized the mysterious deaths were caused by Ebola.

PUBLIC REACTION AFTER EBOLA VIRUS DISEASE OUTBREAK

The reaction of the public changed abruptly when the unnamed disease was eventually declared as Ebola by the Ministry of Health and Social Welfare of Liberia and the World Health Organization. The announcement resulted in drastic changes in the way people, including health workers, interacted with each other, especially EVD patients and their caregivers (Data Display: GRACE M05AC). As stated earlier, there was paralyzing fear resulting in ostracism and stigmatization in the entire spectrum of community life as shown in the following data display.

IGNORANCE, MISCONCEPTIONS, AND LACK OF KNOWLEDGE ABOUT EBOLA VIRUS DISEASE

The hostile reaction by community members towards survivors and caregivers appears to have been fueled by their ignorance about EVD, especially the mode of transmission. Participants reported that this antisocial reaction could in part be explained by the fact that EVD was a strange disease. Most people lacked knowledge about it, including how the disease was transmitted (Data Display: GRACE M01GO). Since little was known about EVD, it was easy for it to appear strange, which fueled misconceptions about the unknown illness. "Part of the reason why I was labeled dangerous to mingle with was due to the strange nature of Ebola, and the fact that people didn't know and many still don't know much about Ebola. Some thought the disease was like flu, malaria, or HIV; we were stigmatized and isolated" (Data Display: GRACE F7SUV).

- "Community members changed their ways toward us because we were considered dangerous to mingle. I think the reason was that Ebola was a strange disease and most people lack knowledge about it, including how the disease was spread" (Data Display: GRACE F11SUV).
- "I got to realized that one of the reasons people ran away from us was because they did not know the mode of transmission of Ebola. Some people thought it was airborne, so they feared, that is why they were stoning my goats and chickens" (Data Display: GRACE M15SUV).

Hewlett and Hewlett (2005) states that ignorance and lack of understanding during an epidemic contribute significantly to towards fear, ostracism, and stigma. They contended that ignorance could easily lead to misconception and misinformation about a disease which may result in panic and stigma. During panic and ostracism, the health-seeking behavior may be negatively affected which may reduce chances of early detection and treatment, thus influencing the spread of the disease (Chowell & Nishiura, 2014). An incidence of ignorance induced fear and panic occurred in Monrovia during the 2014 EVD outbreak which resulted in so many people fleeing the city, including health workers and government officials (Chan, 2014). Participants reported that when it was known that there was no cure for the disease, and health workers were struggling to develop a control mechanism to contain the spread of the disease; the public panic and fear significantly (Data Display: GRACE M28AC).

Table 7

Theme 5: Surviving Ebola Virus Disease: Implications for Survivors and Caregivers

Summary
1. The experience of surviving EVD (Data Display: GRACE M05AC; GRACE M10SUV).
(a) Physical implications of surviving (Data Display: GRACE F29NG; GRACE F12SUV).
(b) Psychological implications of surviving (Data Display: GRACE M16SUV; GRACE M8SUV).
(c) Social implications of surviving EVD (Data Display: GRACE F6SUV; GRACE M8SUV).
(d) Spiritual implications of surviving EVD (Data Display: GRACE F7SUV; GRACE M13SUV).

(e)   Economic implications of surviving (Data Display: GRACE F11SUV; GRACE F27ME).

Note: Theme and categories developed from data analysis.

THE EXPERIENCE OF SURVIVING EBOLA VIRUS DISEASE

Surviving EVD is certainly associated with several psychological consequences. As explained by Finch (2004), after experiencing a traumatic event, most people get preoccupied for a while with memories of the traumatic event as a way of modifying the painful memories to increase their tolerance. And as time goes on, it is expected that these painful memories should disappear. The survivor then adapts and integrates and finally emerges stronger to face other challenges (Lazarus & Folkman, 1984).

The findings show that for some, surviving EVD was unexpected as a sort of miracle. They felt re-born, signaling the beginning of a gradual and steady return of hope and confidence (Data Display: GRACE M05AC). "I counted each day as the day come and go. After 30 days and I have not yet died, I became to realize that God was on my side. When they re-tested my blood, and the results were negative, I said God is good. I became happy, and I gained courage. My worries began to reduce knowing that I am a survivor. The news gave me confidence" (Data Display: GRACE M10SUV). Still, for another group of participants, the initial news of surviving EVD was received with disbelief. They were unsure that they survived the illness. As caregivers, we were waiting for our time to come, to get sick and die (Data Display: GRACE M20FCG). These verbatim quotes reveal survival experience was commonly unexpected and resulted in a myriad of positive feelings including excitement, hope, and thankfulness. On the other hand, some survivors expressed skepticism and reservation about their survival from EVD as highlighted in the following verbatim quotes.

- "As days passed on and I was not dying, I began to feel good. I became increasingly confident about my survival since I realized that I had spent several days past the expected days to live. I noticed I was regaining strength and my health was improving. I knew I was never going to die" (Data Display: GRACE F14SUV).

- "When they said that my blood test was negative, I couldn't believe it. I was filled with doubt deep down in my heart. I thought they were wrong and the result was not mine, especially just a few days ago my blood test result was positive. Even then there was no specific medicine they had given me to say that I have been cured with that medication" (Data Display: GRACE F12SUV).

PHYSICAL IMPLICATIONS OF SURVIVING EBOLA VIRUS DISEASE

The findings show that the physical consequences of EVD such as body weakness, memory loss, and bladder weakness imposed on survivors were experienced as stressful. It often caused elicit deep emotional reactions from the affected especially when survivors feel that they are being stigmatized and blamed for the weaknesses for which they are held culpable (Data Display: GRACE F29NG).

- "The illness left me with many health problems; I was still not well enough to be discharged, but it was better getting out of here. I was advised to see a physician for nearly everything on me, from my bladder to memory loss" (Data Display: GRACE F6SUV).
- "As I recovered, I needed to see a physician concerning my new condition of forgetfulness, urinary frequency, and uterine growths. I also had to see a gynecologist because I lost my menstrual periods" (Data Display: GRACE F12SUV). De Roo et al., (1995) documented that for survivors, the return of normal body functioning during the recovery period is a very slow and striking experience.

PSYCHOLOGICAL IMPLICATIONS OF SURVIVING EBOLA VIRUS DISEASE

Participants reported that they experienced psychological symptoms of fear, depression, hopelessness, pain, altered body image, and weakness as highlighted in the following verbatim quotes.

- "I cannot stop crying whenever I am reminded of Ebola. Recalling my experience with Ebola stresses me. Thinking of the way the illness treated me, it pains me a lot because I am no longer the way I used to look. The illness left me with many weaknesses" (Data Display: GRACE M16SUV).

- "When I think about Ebola, I get reminded of my days in the isolation ward, when all I thought about was death. I did not have any hope that I could survive the illness" (Data Display: GRACE M8SUV).

SOCIAL IMPLICATIONS OF SURVIVING EBOLA VIRUS DISEASE

Participants reported that in addition to the physical and psychological implications of surviving EVD, other incidences also negatively affected their relationship with community members. A critical social outcome of surviving EVD is that it changed how people related to survivors and caregivers, as this participant put it: "When I came back from the isolation center after surviving Ebola, the people never used to come close to me or neither come to my home. Presently, many of my old friends and neighbors continue to avoid me" (Data Display: GRACE F6SUV). The verbatim quotes below outlined some of the social stigma experienced by survivors and caregivers.

- "The five family members I took care of all died. So when my neighbors heard of these deaths, they feared my remaining family members and me. We were isolated and quarantined. Even when Liberia was declared Ebola-free, my children were not allowed back to school" (Data Display: GRACE F17FCG).
- "We were treated so badly by community members. Overwhelmed by fear and anxiety, no one could come to help us. They ran away from us as we cried for help" (Data Display: GRACE M8SUV).

Hewlett and Amola (2003) documented in their 2000/2001 EVD outbreak in Uganda that individuals and their families who were infected with EVD were subject to ostracism, isolation, and open rejection. Participants reported that as the epidemic ravaged on, they that infected with the disease along with their caregivers were forcibly quarantined by community members. At some point in time, the community members threatened to use violence against them, including stoning to stop them from walking in the streets (Data Display: GRACE M28AC).

SPIRITUAL IMPLICATIONS OF SURVIVING EBOLA VIRUS DISEASE

Participants reported that in addition to the physical, psychological, and social effects of experiencing and coping with the threat of EVD, they also expressed the spiritual dimension of their experience. Most of the participants believed that by surpassing the EVD experience were a manifestation of "still having to complete one's mission on earth," which stems from the belief of "being left by God to fulfill their mission." (Data Display: GRACE F7SUV). Some survivors also believed that survival is a "reward" by God for their diligent service to humanity before eventually dying (Data Display: GRACE M13SUV). Findings of this study show that the role of spirituality and religiosity is cardinal in helping the affected to appreciate and cope with traumatic events.

Participants reported that praying and fervently believing in God propelled them in their journey to overcome the disease (Data Display: GRACE M28AC).

ECONOMIC IMPLICATIONS OF SURVIVING EBOLA VIRUS DISEASE

Participants reported that surviving from EVD and going back to work or getting a new job was a challenge they faced and continue to face. They indicated that for some of them who had businesses such as shops or selling in marketplaces, it was hard to continue doing their businesses because they were labeled as "Ebola-people" (Data Display: GRACE F11SUV). Some of them reported weaknesses and memory loss which impacted their ability to do business, resume their jobs, or get a new job. Survivors and caregivers faced and continued to face challenges of reintegrating into their communities after they became outcasts and expelled from homes. Their clothes and properties were burnt, and the possibility of finding jobs or doing business vanished (Data Display: GRACE F27ME).

One of the factors that exacerbated the economic challenges for survivors and caregivers was the increased orphan burden due to the demise of close relatives. Survivors and caregivers had to meet the financial obligations of deceased family members' children. These financial obligations include schools fees, medical bills, and household needs. All of these challenges became too heavy to bear, as this participant affirmed: "The Ebola outbreak has numerous problems for me. One of the most pressing issues I am currently facing is that of orphans. These children were left by my sisters, brothers, uncles, and aunties after they died from Ebola. It is now my responsibility to take care of them and providing their needs is overwhelming" (Data Display: GRACE F18FCG).

The findings show that survivors and caregivers lost property due to the impact of the epidemic on their lives. The loss from surveillance action was inflicted when volunteers working with the health teams upon reaching the home of EVD patients or contacts, or suspects gathered and burnt their personal belongings such as beddings, clothes, and household items for fear the items would harbor the EVD. "As a survivor, the experience made me lose personal belongings. Some of my properties were destroyed because of being sprayed upon, while the community authority burned others for fear of being infected with Ebola. My goods were banned from being sold to the public, and at one time some volunteers from the Ebola Alert Team came and burnt all my goods" (Data Display: GRACE F11SUV).

Survivors and caregivers reported that after the epidemic, the government or NGOs did not compensate them for lost or damaged belongings. One participant explained that this anomaly created a severe financial burden on her, for which she is not prepared to bear. "The false news of my death was particularly a great blow for me. The news caused me to lose my customers. My saloon had graffiti messages such as "RIP," "Ebola kills" and the saloon was sprayed in and out. Most of my customers thought I was dead" (Data Display: GRACE F12SUV).

COSTLY HEALTH CHECK-UPS AND TREATMENT

Costly health checks were another economic consequence reported by survivors. Survivors explained that while in isolation, all their health checks and treatment costs were covered by the NGOs. When they recovered from the disease, health check-ups and treatment became their responsibility, which is very costly and hard to afford (Data Display: GRACE F30NG). The public health facilities are poorly equipped and lack staff to perform the necessary health check-ups and treatment, leaving them with no alternative but to go to private health facilities which are very costly. The verbatim quotes below highlights survivors struggle to follow up on their treatments.

- "I am worried about my financial ability each time I have to go for a check-up. I need to see a physician concerning issues about my forgetfulness, urinary, frequency, and uterine growths. My husband always had to take a loan to pay for my check-ups and treatment. He is still paying for loans he took in the past to pay for my treatment. I told him to sell our land so that we can use the money for check-ups, treatment, and good food to recover quickly" (Data Display: GRACE F14SUV).

- "I am worried about my financial ability each time I have to go for a check-up. I need to see a physician concerning issues about my forget-fulness, urinary, frequency, and uterine growths. My husband always had to take a loan to pay for my check-ups and treatment. He is still paying for loans he took in the past to pay for my treatment. I told him to sell our land so that we can use the money for check-ups, treatment, and good food to recover quickly" (Data Display: GRACE F14SUV).

These verbatim expressions signal the presence of financial stress participants experienced, especially survivors who had to undergo these expensive treatments and health check-ups. The study shows that the financial crises are because survivors have reduced opportunities to work or do businesses due to the widespread rejection and discrimination melted on them by society. The study also show that survivors were limited to get jobs or to do businesses due to their new health conditions such as reduced physical and mental capacity to perform their duties.

SUMMARY

During the study, there was no discrepancy in literature or findings. Chapter 4 introduced the following five themes: (1) Descriptive overview of coping with the threat of EVD, (2) Social-cultural beliefs, practices, and economic factors related to EVD, (3) Nature of EVD experience, (4) Reactions towards EVD outbreak, and (5) Surviving EVD: implications for survivors and caregivers. These themes were perceived from the face-to-face interviews with 30 EVD participants in Monrovia. The interviews primarily focused on coping with the threat of Ebola, the role of the caring others, and the reactions of the general public towards EVD survivors and their family caregivers. The chapter also explained the process of how the data were analyzed, as well as how the five themes and categories were recognized.

The goal of understanding the EVD survivors' and their family caregivers' experiences in relationship to Ebola, the public reactions, and their cultural and religious beliefs was achieved. The following research questions were answered.

Question 1: How did survivors and family caregivers cope with the threat of EVD in Monrovia in 2014? Each EVD survivor and their family caregiver interviewed expressed some form of stigmatization, ostracism, and rejection by family, friends, and the public. Survivors explained that their survival was a blessing from God because no health worker could guarantee their chances of surviving EVD. Caregivers demonstrated love for loved ones by staying with them in such difficult time. They too explained that being kept safe from contracting EVD was a divine act of God so that they could stay alive to provide care for their loved ones.

Question 2: What social, cultural and economic factors may have contributed to the spread of EVD in Monrovia in 2014? All participants expressed that the spread of EVD was due to social, cultural and economic factors. They explained that it was difficult for them to abandon their life-long cultural practices of taking care of their sick relatives or burial rites as means to contain the spread of EVD. Poverty was another factor expressed by participants that influenced the spread of EVD. People were compared to leave their homes and go fetch for food or jobs to sustain their families. This situation caused fluid population movement thus fueling the rapid spread of EVD.

Question 3: How did government policies of mandatory cremation and banning of public gathering impact the containment of EVD in Monrovia in 2014? The Liberian government in an effort to contain the spread of EVD, ban public gathering including the closing of schools and offices. Participants expressed that the ban was implemented without public assistant such food and water to support residents to stay indoors. There was a public outcry when traditional burial practices were halted and replaced by cremation EVD victims without the participation of relatives. Question 4: What social stigma did EVD impact on survivors?

EVD survivors expressed that they were and continue to be discriminated in society due to the stigma of EVD. They explained that people are reluctant to interact with them. Returning to their market stall or place of work has been challenging because people consider them dangerous to mingle with.

In Chapter 5, the five themes are discussed based on the semi-structured interviews with the 30 research participants. These discussions are in relationship to the research literature through a realistic and comprehensive portrait of the phenomenon using stories of all participants. Chapter 5 highlights the implications and limitations of the study followed by the researcher's plan of action for creating positive social change, recommendations for future practice, summary and conclusions of the study.

CHAPTER 5

DISCUSSION, CONCLUSIONS, AND RECOMMENDATIONS

INTRODUCTION

In this final chapter, the research process was summarized, highlighting each of the five themes key interpretations of findings, conclusions, and recommendations. The study's limitations and implication for social and policy change were also discussed. The discussions on the five themes including categories as explicated in Chapter 4 were explained within the selected theoretical framework to demonstrate their trustworthiness. The Bandura SCT framework employed for this study suggested a theory of human motivation and action from a social cognitive perspective.

Bandura (1997) stressed that the application of observational learning, imitation, and modeling integrates a continuous interaction between behaviors, personal factors, cognition, and the environment. Behavior refers to the complexity and skills, among others, related to an individual. The environment refers to where the phenomenon occurred and it describes the situation, roles, models, and the relationships. A personal factor (person) refers to cognition which describes self-efficacy, motives, and personality. The SCT served as the guiding theoretical framework for this study which was applied throughout this research. I hoped to have generated accurate, reliable, and productive and reproducible data, through interviews, observations, documentation, and analyses, to increase the body of knowledge (Merriam, 2009) relevant to the phenomenon for further discussion among community members, health workers, leaders, and policymakers.

The purpose of this qualitative case study was to explore the social, economic, and policy factors that contributed to the spread of the 2014 EVD outbreak in Liberia. I designed this study to gain a clear understanding of how people experienced the phenomenon of coping with the threat of EVD. Especially, how the public perceived EVD and the change in attitudes of survivors. Further, what the public reactions towards EVD symbolized, including their reactions towards persons and families affected by EVD.

The nature of the study included a qualitative case study inquiry that facilitated data collection through interviews, observations, documentation, and tape-recordings to serve the study's purpose to explore the potential of how residents of Monrovia coped with the threat of EVD. Key findings, creating evidence of value (Campbell, 2014) included verbatim quotes from participants expressing their experiences of how they coped with the threat of EVD. Participants expressed the need for government, policymakers, and nongovernmental organizations to develop comprehensive intervention techniques, disease awareness education, financial assistance for survivors, and a cure for EVD.

INTERPRETATIONS OF THE FINDINGS

In this section, I summarized salient features of the study, namely themes and categories which included the all-encompassing concept of adaptation. Informed by the interpretation of findings for each of the five themes, I made pertinent conclusions and recommendations for this study.

THEME 1: DESCRIPTIVE OVERVIEW OF COPING WITH THREAT OF EVD

Findings. Participants in this study described coping with the threat of EVD as terrifying. They expressed numerous negative experiences including coming face-to-face with death. Survivors and caregivers reported experiencing intense fear, ostracism, and stigmatization (Data Display: GRACE M05AC; GRACE F6SUV). They felt that EVD had annihilated them from their existence and diminished their possibilities (Data Display: GRACE M05AC). Survivors and caregivers explained that a defining feature of the traumatic experience was that the negative experiences such as social isolation lingered on for several months even after they were declared Ebola-free, and the when the epidemic came to an end (Data Display: GRACE F6SUV; GRACE F17FCG).

These actions resulted in several psychosomatic manifestations during and after the EVD outbreak (Data Display: GRACE F12SUV; GRACE F19FCG). Participants and community members concluded that suffering from EVD was an inescapable reality (Data Display: GRACE M8SUV; GRACE F29NG). The findings also show that even though the outbreak was frightening and traumatic, most survivors and caregivers adapted to the threat and reality of EVD by actively seeking opportunities for self-preservation and protection. These actions helped the majority of them to transcend their victimhood state and became empowered individuals (Data Display: GRACE F7SUV).

Conclusions. Living in an EVD prone area signifies a real threat to one's life especially during an epidemic. Evidence in the study shows that when such an outbreak occurs, the experience is not only terrifying, but it is life-threatening as well. The situation creates the possibility of death due to the high virulence of EVD. The findings further indicated that if the appropriate and timely interventions are not implemented, the widespread fear, ostracism, and stigmatization could proliferate to disproportionate levels leading to the severe annihilation of survivors and caregivers.

Additionally, this could limit their opportunities for meaningful living within the short and long term, by implying a potentially negative effect on their wellbeing. The findings also indicated that while EVD is experienced as traumatic, survivors and caregivers' adaptive capacity played a necessary role in mediating these negative experiences. Their role in their self-preservation and protection efforts, including their journeys of transcending from being helpless victims to becoming empowered members of the community, demonstrated their adaptive capacities.

Recommendations. The following recommendations were made to reduce fear, ostracism, and stigmatization and the resulting disproportionate annihilation of survivors and caregivers in the future. It is recommended that during outbreaks, continuous education of the public should be carried out by the government, health workers, and trained community volunteers using radios and through home visits. The disease education effort should be focused on the signs and symptoms of EVD, procedures for protecting family members as well as appropriate referral including an expectation of antisocial behavior. The role of the media should include educating the public about the etiological aspect of the disease to help reduce the anxiety and misinformation commonly associated with EVD outbreaks particularly, the infection and transmission methods. Health authorities must train volunteers, and their mobilization efforts should include the distribution of information, education and communication messages using posters, flyers, and brochures. The education efforts should also include volunteers speaking to community members in their local dialects for easy understanding of the cause, transmission, and prevention techniques of the disease.

This approach was used by the International Federation of Red Cross and Red Crescent Societies during the 2012 EVD outbreak in Uganda, and it resulted in considerable reduction of disease transmission and mortalities (IFRC & RC, 2012). It is recommended that government improved their healthcare capacity including infrastructure and trained staff. It is also recommended that those who contract the disease should be handled by trained health workers in a manner that reduces public terror and anxiety. Volunteers should not destroy or burn properties of EVD patients, survivors or caregivers; instead, they should enhance the adaptive capacity of survivors and caregivers by helping them in a holistic manner. Survivors and caregivers should be supported by finding meaning in their experience, to enable them to gain the ability to overcome their new life challenges and as well as restore their self-esteem through positive self-evaluation.

THEME 2: SOCIAL-CULTURAL BELIEFS, PRACTICES, AND ECONOMIC FACTORS RELATED TO EVD

Findings. Participants reported that they understood EVD from two perspectives: either as a supernatural occurrence or as a natural occurrence. Those who perceived EVD as supernatural occurrence as expressed in data display (Data Display: GRACE F26FCG; GRACE M15SUV), attributed the outbreak to Satanic or evil spirits attacks. They believed that the disease is a punishment by deities, and work by enemies of their family. Some regarded the outbreak as the work of witchcraft, charm or sorcery. In contrast, those who believed EVD as a naturally occurring disease as explained in data display (Data Display: GRACE M16SUV; GRACE F26FCG), thought of it as a common infectious disease that spreads through contact from one person to another.

Meanwhile, those who believed EVD is a supernatural occurrence sought supernatural healing remedies from churches, mosques, and healing places, operated by locally revered prophets, prophetesses, and spiritualists.

The study further shows that those who believed EVD as a natural occurrence sought treatment from regular clinics, hospitals, and other health facilities. The study also show a third group of individuals who have tried help from both biomedical sources such as drugs stores, hospitals, and clinics; as well as, from supernatural sources like spiritual healers, prophets, prophetesses, and witchdoctors.

Conclusions. The findings indicate that the community understood EVD as either as a supernatural or a natural occurring inflicted disease. These beliefs influenced their choices of treatment, depending on whether they perceived EVD as a supernatural occurrence associated with spiritual powers, or as a common infectious disease requiring biomedical interventions. These actions have grave implications for disease control because health seeking patterns were determined by the individual's perception of what causes EVD. For health workers and policymakers to ensure success in future epidemics, it is critical to understand the perspectives individuals hold about the causes of EVD, as this directly influences their health seeking practices.

Recommendations. Informed by these findings, it is recommended that during the early days of an epidemic, the etiological models of EVD need to be identified to perform suitable intervention techniques that can counter negative perceptions. In the same vein, by encouraging those perspectives that contribute positively towards containing the outbreak. These recommendations are consistent with Helman's (2007) "culture, health, and illness." Helman affirmed that due to the complex nature of human relationships and especially how people are intricately influenced by their backgrounds, a person's culture is often the inherited habit in which he or she perceives and understands the world. Helman stressed that in situations such as EVD outbreaks, people respond differently, some will turn to their natural environment, and others will turn to supernatural forces for cure or healing. He noted that because of the great importance culture plays in ones live; it is crucial to understanding the socio-cultural dimensions underlying people's health values, beliefs, and behaviors. Helman (2007) further stressed that this practice would ensure successful patient clinical outcomes during disease outbreaks such as EVD.

This recommendation is also consistent with Chowell & Nishiura's (2014) "transmission dynamics and control of ebola virus disease" models of care and treatment, where healthcare workers (caregivers) are required to work with recipients of care to preserve positive health practices and values. It is also recommended that survivors and caregivers' cultural beliefs and values be respected to ensure that the health messages and disease education information packages are evidence-based and is culturally-sensitive. These messages should address those concerns that are counterproductive to epidemic response efforts, thereby increasing chances of being accepted. Understanding the dominant explanatory models also promotes identification of key stakeholders such as prophets, prophetesses, and spiritualists, who can become the point of contacts for the community to facilitate the encouragement of early and timely referral of patients to established treatment centers. This recommendation can serve as a recognition and collaboration that can limit the spread of EVD due to early case detection leading to timely and proper isolation of infected individuals.

THEME 3: NATURE OF EBOLA VIRUS DISEASE EXPERIENCE

Findings. The study shows that participants experienced the EVD outbreak as both a positive and negative event, with the experience defined by the central role caring others played in their struggle to survive (Data Display: GRACE M24FCG; GRACE F30NG). The findings also indicate that survivors and caregivers vacillated between episodes of hope and hopelessness (Data Display: GRACE F12SUV; GRACE M22FCG) during the outbreak period and even in the aftermath. It was discovered that survivors and caregivers had both positive and negative experiences. The positive outcomes relate to improvements in personal hygiene and protection practices (Data Display: GRACE F26FCG; GRACE M04NG). Self-awareness and health seeking behavior (Data Display: GRACE F30NG; GRACE M09ME); as well as improved clinical care practices (Data Display: GRACE M25FCG; GRACE M16SUV).

The findings show that negative outcomes were the abandonment of culturally cherished practices of congeniality (Data Display: GRACE M15SUV; GRACE M14SUV), loss of close relatives (Data Display: GRACE F12SUV; GRACE F6SUV), ceaseless rejection of survivors and caregivers (Data Display: GRACE M10SUV; GRACE M17SUV), widespread isolation and ostracism (Data Display: GRACE M10SUV); as well as stigmatization, shame, and embarrassment (Data Display: GRACE M17SUV).

Conclusions. The findings indicate that experiencing an EVD outbreak has both positive and negative consequences. The findings also show that the role of caring others, either as relatives, health workers, or volunteers helped survivors to adapt to the negative effects of EVD. It is evident that experiencing EVD is associated with episodes of optimism for favorable outcomes at one time and experience of hopelessness and despair at another. It is also evident from the study that, while EVD outbreaks are mostly dreaded, they can still have positive outcomes.

For example, the EVD outbreak taught survivors and caregivers personal hygiene and self-protection practices and increased their self-awareness. It also taught them health seeking behavior, particularly in the aftermath of the outbreak. The findings also show that the EVD outbreak resulted in improved clinical and healthcare practices of survivors and caregivers, especially among healthcare workers. From a negative aspect, the unprecedented deaths exacerbated abandonment of culturally cherished practices of congeniality leading to isolation, ostracism, and stigmatization of survivors, caregivers, and close associates.

Recommendations. Cognizant that an EVD outbreak has both positive and negative outcomes for survivors and caregivers, it is recommended that appropriate interventions techniques be devised to exploit the central role of the caring others. In this regard, it will assist survivors and caregivers in their struggle against the undesirable consequences of the epidemic. Communities should be educated through social health education campaigns during and in between an outbreak. Accomplishing this can be done by using different media sources designed to support individuals and families affected by EVD, especially, after they are declared Ebola-free. It is further recommended that in Ebola prone areas, the Ministry of Health should foster continuing health education (epidemic) program for personal hygiene and protection practices to increase self-awareness and health seeking behavior. Participants in such health education program should be awarded "certificates of cleanliness" by health authorities.

The Ministry of Health through NGOs and other local agencies should also develop health education programs in local dialects to help reduce the unprecedented fear caused by misinformation and exaggeration about EVD. To ensure culturally congruent care, it is recommended that during outbreaks, there is need to uphold one of the most sacred ceremonies highly valued by locals. The burial team should work hand-in-hand with locals or especially one influential (designated) member of the family to conduct some basic burial ritual while wearing protective clothing. This practice will help to dignify the dead and make the family feel inclusive in the home going of their loved one. Farmer (2001) described this culture care preservation model of healthcare which means to provide congruent health; professional caregivers should uphold patients' cultural practices and beliefs as long as they promote their recovery. Tosh and Sampathkumar (2014) affirmed that such therapeutic care modes fit with people's ways of life, and satisfy them, leading to better cooperation.

THEME 4: REACTIONS TOWARDS EBOLA VIRUS DISEASE OUTBREAK

Findings. The findings show that before the 2014 EVD outbreak, communities in Monrovia were well integrated. These communities were socially vibrant, and individuals and families carried out routine activities including trade and work (Data Display: GRACE F27ME; GRACE M28AC). But when EVD was confirmed, it provoked fear, panic, and ostracism which resulted in creating widespread stigmatization of infected individuals and their families (Data Display: GRACE M05AC). The hysteria was exacerbated by unsubstantiated media reports that amplified the ferocity of the disease; leading to the abandonment of key culturally cherished practices of congeniality.

Conclusions. The findings indicate that the advent of EVD disturbed the traditional social platform of the community. As a result, it created the emergence of antisocial acts of ostracism and stigmatization due to pervasive fear and panic associated with the EVD outbreak. These antisocial reactions appeared to have fueled by ignorance and misconceptions about EVD. The findings show that the need for continuous health (disease) education was necessary. The media should play a vital role in educating the public about the actual cause of EVD, including how it is transmitted, its accurate picture and how to prevent it from spreading to others. Health education is crucial because fear and hysteria seem to arise from people's desire to protect themselves from the actual and exaggerated dangers of EVD outbreaks.

Recommendations. For future outbreaks, it is recommended that interventions should focus on maintaining the integrity of the community members. Maintaining their integrity will increase their resilience to the upsetting nature of EVD. Community members should receive accurate information about EVD, including its manner of transmission and prevention to minimize the fear and hysteria that commonly surrounds outbreaks. The early integration of the media is critical to ensure accurate and responsible reporting, because unconfirmed reporting inadvertently amplifies outbreaks, leading to an extraordinary social frenzy. It is also recommended that such interventions should start as soon as an outbreak is declared, and should continue long into the aftermath. The media should work in collaboration with health workers to first understand the etiology of the epidemic; this will ensure that the public is provided with accurate information. Doing this will reduce the widespread misinformation and exaggeration commonly associated with outbreaks.

These recommendations are consistent with Tosh and Sampathkumar (2014) stating that it is critical to understand the unending risks of transmission dynamics and resurgence of EVD. Community mistrust challenges social mobilization and community health education during epidemics of high mortality. The first thing to do in this situation is trying to get the communities to accept the illness and the necessities for clinical care. Ensuring this understanding will help in implementing rapid and efficient response interventions designed to specific local settings and context. Community understanding of the clinical presentation, clinical course, transmission, and prevention of EVD can help reduce anxiety, panic, and stigma associated with the disease and allow healthcare providers to provide medical care to individuals suspected of having EVD confidently.

Leroy et al. (2005) suggested that in the absence of an effective primary prevention technique, the central epidemic management should rely on educating the communities about EVD. During EVD outbreaks, traditional practices such as burial rites should be suspended and enforced in agreement with those who practice these rituals. IFRC and RCS (2012) stated that the 2000-2001 EVD outbreaks in Gulu, Uganda was significantly contained with the help of social mobilization. De Roo et al. (1995) confirmed that EVD awareness and education through the media or local cultural performances (drama groups) designed to win the confidence and support of rural residents must first be put into effect while awaiting the invention of EVD vaccines and or cure. WHO (2014) agreed that the use of media including documentary films would enhance epidemic preparedness and response.

THEME 5: SURVIVING EVD: IMPLICATIONS FOR SURVIVORS AND CAREGIVERS

Findings. Surviving EVD has an overwhelming effect on the well-being of survivors and caregivers, which may be categorized as physical (Data Display: GRACE F29NG; GRACE F12SUV), psychological (Data Display: GRACE M16SUV; GRACE M8SUV), social (Data Display: GRACE M16SUV; GRACE M8SUV), spiritual (Data Display: GRACE M13SUV GRACE M8SUV) and as well as economic (Data Display: GRACE F11SUV; GRACE F27ME). The physical consequences included body weakness, pain, loss of memory and bladder weakness, these affected survivors' physical integrity and self-esteem. The psychological effects were fear, depression, hopelessness, pain altered body image and numbness.

Socially, there were reports of protracted ostracism, rejection, and stigmatization. Spiritually, the findings show that the participants experienced increased sense of religiosity and the feeling that their survival meant they still had to "complete their mission on earth." Others attributed their survival to "reward" from God (Data Display: GRACE M13SUV GRACE M8SUV). The economic implications undoubtedly arose out of increased expenditure due to loss of properties, loss of businesses, and loss of jobs caused community reactions towards survivors and caregivers. Costly medical treatments as well as loss of income arising out of the inability for survivors and caregivers to work due to weakness and memory loss, and social stigma and rejection.

Conclusions. The news of surviving EVD was experienced as delightful. Most survivors considered it as "the impossible becoming a reality." However, survival resulted in several repercussions within physical, psychological, social, spiritual, and economic realms. These experiences negatively affected the survivors' well-being and precipitated poorer health outcomes. These experiences call for resilience building during and in between EVD outbreaks.

Recommendations. The Ministry of Health should improve its public health facilities to include specialized clinics for treating EVD and making follow-ups of survivors. Doing this will address the physical and mental health needs of survivors, and help to contain the spread of EVD during future outbreaks. It is further recommended that during these clinic visits, survivors and their family members should receive psychotherapy sessions to address psychological challenges the disease may have impacted on them. These sessions should also address the root causes of their rejection and stigmatization experienced by survivors and caregivers.

It is also recommended that the Ministry of Health in collaboration with the Ministry of Information should develop appropriate guidelines for disseminating messages related to epidemic broadcast by the media. Ensuring these guidelines will promote responsible journalism and help to reduce the fear and panic associated with outbreaks. The health authorities should closely monitor the media and support their work by involving them early in the epidemic response efforts. Health officials should provide accurate information about the disease to the media for onward dissemination to the public. These accurate health education messages would help minimize the widespread hysteria and anxiety associated with EVD. Continuing mass health education using radio, print, and electronic mediums would address the social aspect of the outbreak, including isolation and stigmatization of survivors and caregivers. The health education efforts should also include a house-to-house health promotion visits in all communities.

These recommendations are consistent with Hodge et al.'s (2014) recommendation that EVD-affected countries should evaluate and intensify their respective national public health emergency preparedness and response plans and national command and coordination structures. Accomplishing this task requires health officials adapt an incident management structure (IMS) and emergency operations center (EOC) to reinforce emergency health operations. It is also recommended that upon surviving EVD, the survivor should be discharged and escorted home along with an official from the Ministry of Health to hand them officially to their family and community with a "certificate" that they are declared Ebola-free. Doing this would assure the family and the community that the survivor is no longer infectious, and should be allowed to re-integrate into the community freely.

Spiritually, survivors and caregivers should be encouraged to continue to uphold their religious beliefs; so long it does not interfere with compromise infection control efforts. Helman (2007) states that in situations such as EVD outbreaks, people respond differently, some will turn to their natural environment, and others will turn to supernatural forces for cure or healing. Hewlett and Amola (2003) noted that not all traditional healers could heal EVD and other related diseases because they have to encounter the spirits and the spirits are too strong to face.

LIMITATIONS OF THE STUDY

In spite of the fact that the study produced credible information about the lived experiences of EVD survivors and their caregivers, it also inevitably has some limitations. The following are some of the limitations in the study: This study used a qualitative research design; this means that the study documented the experience of a comparatively limited number of participants. In most cases, this has an adverse bearing on the generalizability of the study findings to other settings; which would have been different if the study was quantitative in its approach. Limitations of this study could be due to the responses of participants that could be skewed due to respondents' bias. Data for this study primarily depended on interviews which were self-reported. Self-reporting is not always reliable because an individual may provide an answer he or she thinks is correct as opposed to what he or she genuinely feels. This bias could diminish the validity of the data.

Another limitation of this study was time. This study explored all avenues to ensure that more time was available for interviews, observations, and documentation of participants. The context-specific nature of the study means that analysis and the interpretation of the research data depended on the researcher's choices. The same data could have been interpreted differently by another researcher and could have potentially led to different findings.

Despite these limitations, the findings are reliable, valid, and trustworthy. Especially, given that the data collection and analysis methods utilized were thorough. Pre-testing of the interview questions was conducted to ensure the validity of the study's instrument. The instrument was valid and it measured what it was supposed to measure to attain reliability and validity. The researcher ensured that the transition from raw data to informed data was valid. Trustworthiness in this study was achieved because there was confidence in the truth of the findings and also because the findings has applicability in other contexts. The findings in this study were consistent and it can be repeated. The findings further demonstrated a degree of neutrality because the study was shaped by the respondents and not researcher's bias, motivation, or interest. Credibility of the research findings was established through prolonged engagement with research participants which included the incorporation of method and data triangulation. The researcher spent sufficient time with each participant and during this process; accurate and rich data were obtained to understand the phenomenon better. The prolonged engagement was fortified with some follow-ups interviews.

The findings present valuable insight suggesting that survivors and caregivers admitted their actual experiences as it relates to EVD. The study shows evidence where many of the survivors and caregivers adjusted to their new lives. Some even thrived by experiencing personal growth within the context of psychological support they received from family members and friends. The knowledge gained is thus enlightening since it has humbly contributed to a deeper understanding of how the survivors, caregivers, and the general public experienced EVD during and after the EVD outbreak.

RECOMMENDATIONS FOR FUTURE RESEARCH

The findings of this study suggested the need for further research to be conducted to understand the followings: To understand the views and ideas of community members, including health workers, spouses of EVD victims and survivors, and orphans. Also widows/widowers and children of survivors/victims. Survivors should be explored to get a holistic picture of the concept of resilience within these groups. It is recommended that further research design to incorporate a larger sample of participants from various parts of the country including communities that were not hit by the EVD epidemic. Such research would help widen and gain a broader understanding of how people perceive EVD from the current study.

Further studies should be conducted to explore the experiences of survivors and caregivers, in the long run, to understand how the concept of resilience evolves over time. To investigate the associated social-cultural variables to understand how affected individuals modify the EVD experience during and after the outbreak. It is recommended that a study is conducted that emphasizes community empowerment as it relates to the fear, stigma, and ostracism associated with EVD. It is recommended that the concept of adaptation among EVD survivors and caregivers be further explained as a multidimensional and multifaceted concept. Doing this could create the possibility of developing a conceptual system that could be used to enhance the adaptive capacity of survivors and caregivers including people who may become affected by EVD in the future.

IMPLICATIONS FOR SOCIAL AND POLICY CHANGE

Since the initial outbreaks of EVD in the DRC and Sudan in 1976, healthcare practitioners have been challenged to contain EVD, thus posing a global threat of spreading the disease. This study hopes to make an original contribution by improving on the knowledge gap in the literature geared to creating an efficient mechanism to contain EVD, which will add to the existing knowledge that key policymakers and health practitioners rely upon to make decisions. In this study, factors that influenced the abandonment and rejection, isolation and ostracism, and stigmatization of EVD survivors and caregivers were identified.

These findings, if implemented, would help in educating individuals, families, community members and the general public in treating and accepting especially EVD survivors as heroes and not as victims or dangerous individuals in the community. This study used a case study methodology to investigate the lived experiences of EVD survivors, family caregivers, NGO staff, government officials, academicians, and members from the media who were directly involved in the 2014 EVD outbreak. The study findings, when used, may strengthen decision-making and policy guidelines always to involve the media from the beginning of the outbreak to ensure accurate reporting about the etiological aspect of the epidemic. Also, health workers, policymakers, and the community members should work in collaboration to contain the spread and transmission of EVD. It is also anticipated that this study may contribute to positive social change by improving policies and training practices for healthcare practitioners on appropriate intervention techniques to effectively contain EVD.

Since Liberia has just emerged from a 14 year civil war which devastated its health facilities, this study provides additional information that should support and facilitate improved epidemic intervention strategies when an outbreak occurs. This study may also contribute to community knowledge base towards a better understanding of some of the factors that affect, and or may affect future outbreaks of EVD such as better hygiene practices and the use of PPE by health workers, caregivers and anyone coming across suspected EVD patients. Findings from this study provided relevant, reliable and verifiable information that should guide community members, health workers, and policy makers aimed at improving the relationship with survivors, caregivers, and the community members.

This research study may contribute to positive social and policy change by providing an enhanced understanding of what it is to be affected by EVD. The study explained the experiences of survivors and family caregivers, including officials of government, NGO staff, academicians, and reporters from the media who experienced the outbreak. In this regard, their insight may broaden the public's understanding of what it means to be affected by EVD. This new knowledge may change people's overall perceptions and beliefs about EVD. Community engagement in the implementation of the findings may result in community empowerment and the understanding of coping with the threat of EVD, which may benefit individuals, organizations, and society in general.

Knowledge gained from the findings would empower health workers and policy makers with information for better health programming in Liberia. Findings should serve as baseline information for evidence-based policies, especially in containing the spread and transmission of EVD during outbreaks. The findings in this study generated new understanding of EVD survivors' and family caregivers' experiences of caring for sick relatives and being affected by EVD. Results may provide insight into better policy and epidemic response during future EVD outbreaks. This study also explored the experiences of EVD survivors and family caregivers and provided basis for creating effective policies to contain EVD and better preparation of health care workers during future outbreaks. The findings may contribute towards more comprehensive health care policy changes and protocols that could better address the health needs of the affected patients, the survivors, and society in general.

CONCLUSIONS

This chapter concludes the study. In this section, an overview of the research process is outlined to draw the attention of the reader to the various steps that were used in the study. The main findings were summarized, conclusions were drawn, and key recommendations were made. The recommendations in this study are based on the five themes that emerged from the study. As previously mentioned, this study explored the social, economic and policy-related factors that influenced the spread of the 2014 EVD in Monrovia. Findings from this study generated new understanding of EVD survivors' and caregivers' experiences of caring for sick relatives as well as being affected by EVD. The experiences of EVD survivors, caregivers, health care workers, and policymakers provided a basis for better preparation of all stakeholders and the communities during future outbreaks.

The primary purpose of this study was to gain a clear understanding of how residents of Monrovia experience the phenomenon of coping with the threat of EVD. Especially, how they perceive EVD and the change in attitudes of survivors, what their reactions towards EVD symbolize, including their reactions towards persons and families affected by EVD. The study further explored how governments' decrees and regulations influenced the spread of EVD instead of containing it. The researcher collected data through interviews, observations, documentation, and analyses, to increase the body of knowledge (Merriam, 2009) relevant to the phenomenon for further discussion among community members, health workers, leaders, and policymakers. The researcher hoped to have generated accurate, reliable, and productive and reproducible information that could reduce fear, stigmatization, abandonment, isolation and ostracism during future outbreaks. The need for further research is crucial in addressing the issues of fear, stigma, isolation, abandonment, and ostracism associated with the disease that could allow healthcare providers to confidently provide medical care to individuals suspected of having EVD (Tosh & Sampathkumar, 2014).

Based on the data, the researcher suggested several recommendations for future research. The recommendations include the need to understand the views and ideas of community members, including health workers, spouses of EVD victims and survivors, and orphans. In this vein, survivors and caregivers should be further explored to get a holistic picture of the concept of resilience within these groups. Research should be designed to incorporate a larger sample of participants from various parts of the country including communities that were not hit by the 2014 EVD outbreak. Such research if implemented would help widen and gain a broader understanding of how people perceive EVD from the current study. Also, there are many areas for potential positive social change outlined in the study that could benefit Monrovians and society in general.

Finally, factors that influenced the abandonment, isolation, ostracism, and stigmatization of EVD survivors and caregivers were identified in the study. These findings, if implemented, would help in improving community relationship with survivors and caregivers. The study findings may provide insight so as to strengthen decision-making and policy guidelines that could promote cooperation with EVD patients, survivors, caregivers, health workers, policymakers, and the general public.

REFERENCES

Archibald, C. M., & Newman, D. (2015). Pilot testing HIV prevention in an Afro Caribbean faith-based community. *Association of Black Nursing Faculty Journal, 26(2), 43–49.* Retrieved from http://www.pubfacts.com/detail/26197635/PilotTesting-HIV-Prevention-in-an-Afro-Caribbean-Faith-Based-Community

Bandura, A. (1997). *Self-efficacy: The exercise of control.* New York: Freeman.

Bellizzi, S. (2014). The current ebola outbreak: Old and new contexts. *Journal of Infection in Developing Countries, 8(11), 1378-1380.* doi:10.3855/jidc.6142

Bertaux, D. (1981). *Biography and society: The life history approach in the social sciences.* London: Sage.

Biernacki, P., & Waldorf, D. (1981). *Snowball sampling: Problems and techniques of chain referral sampling.* Retrieved from http://isites.harvard.edu/fs/docs/icb.topic536746.files/Biernacki_Waldorf_Snowball_Sampling.pdf

Centers for Disease Control and Prevention. (2014). *Ebola outbreaks 2000-2014* Retrieved from http://www.cdc.gov/vhf/ebola/outbreaks/history/summaries.html

Chan, M. (2014). Ebola virus disease in West Africa: No early end to the outbreak. *The New England Journal of Medicine, 371,* 1183-1185. doi:10.1056/NEJMp1409859

Charmaz, K. (2006). *Constructing grounded theory: A practical guide through qualitative analysis.* Thousand Oaks, CA: Sage.

Chowell, G., & Nishiura, H. (2014). Transmission dynamics and control of ebola virus disease. *BMC Medicine, 12,* 196. doi:10.1186/s12916-014-0196-0

Damen, L. (1987). *Culture learning: The fifth dimension in the language class-room*. Reading, MA: Addison-Wesley.

De Roo, A., Ado, B., Rose, B., Guimard, Y., Fonck, K., & Colebunders, R. (1995). Survey among survivors of the 1995 ebola epidemic in Kikwit, Democratic Republic of Congo: Their feelings and experiences. *Tropical Medicine and International Health, 3*(11), 883–885. Retrieved from http://web.a.ebscohost.com.ezp.waldenulibrary.org/ehost/pdfviewer/pdfview er ?vi d=34&sid=d5a6efa6-f5d0-4b4f-a599- 4fc9eea39cfe%40sessionmgr4002&hid=4109

Deci, E., & Ryan, R. (2002). *Handbook of self-determination research*. Roches-ter: University of Rochester Press.

Ertmer, P. A., & Ottenbreit-Leftwich, A. T. (2010). Teacher technology change: How knowledge, confidence, beliefs and culture intersect. *JRTE, 42*, 255-284

Farmer, P. (2001). *Infections and inequalities: The modern plagues*. Berkeley: University of California Press.

Feldmann, H., & Geisbert, T. W. (2012). Ebola haemorrhagic fever. *Lancet. 377(9768): 849–862*. doi:10.1016/S0140-6736(10)60667-8

Finch, L. P. (2004). Understanding patients' lived experiences: The inter-relationship of rhetoric and hermeneutics. *Nursing Philosophy, 5*(3), 251-257

Folkman, S., & Lazarus, R. S. (1980). An analysis of coping in a middle-aged community sample. *Journal of Health and Social Behavior*, 21, pp. 219–239

Foster, G. M. (1976). Disease etiologies in non-western medical systems. *American Anthropologist. 78: 773–782*. doi:10.1525/aa.1976.78.4.02a00030

Giorgi, A. (1997). The theory, practice, and evaluation of the phenomeno-logical method as a qualitative research procedure. *Journal of Phenome-nological Psychology, 10*, 1163. doi:10.1163/156916297X00103

Gomes, M. F. C., Pastore y Piontti, A., Rossi, L., Chao, D., Longini, I., Hal-loran, M. E., & Vespignani, A. (2014). Assessing the international spreading risk associated with the 2014 West African ebola outbreak. *PLOS Currents Outbreaks, 1*(10), 1371. doi:10.1371/currents.outbreaks.cd818f63d40e24aef769dda7df9e0da5

Helman, C. G. (2007). *Culture, health and illness* (5th ed.). London: Hodder Arnold. CRC Press LLC.

Hewlett, B. S. & Amola, R. P. (2003). Cultural contexts of ebola in Northern Uganda.

Journal of Infectious Diseases. 9(10): 1242–1248 doi:10.3201/eid0910.020493

Hewlett, B. L., & Hewlett, B. S. (2005). Providing care and facing death: nursing during Ebola outbreaks in central Africa. *Journal of Transcultural Nursing, 16(4), 289-297.*

Hodge, J. G., Barraza, L., Measer, G., & Agrawal, A. (2014). *Global emergency legal responses to the 2014 ebola outbreak: Public health and the law.* Retrieved from http://web.a.ebscohost.com.ezp.waldenulibrary.org/ehost/pdfviewer/pdfviewer?sid=d5a6efa6-f5d0-4b4f-a599-4fc9eea39cfe%40sessionmgr4002&vid=7&hid=4109

Howard, G. S. (1980). *Response-shift bias: A problem in evaluating interventions with pre/post self-reports.* Retrieved from http://www.jae-online.org/attachments/article/463/40-04-28.pdf

Howe H., Lake A., & Shen, T. (2007). Method to assess identifiability in electronic data files. *American Journal of Epidemiology*, 165, 597–60. doi:10.1177/10497323093 50879

International Federation of Red Cross & Red Crescent Societies. (2012). *Uganda: Ebola outbreak.* Retrieved from http://www.ifrc.org/docs/Appeals/12/MDRUG031fr.pdf

Jerving, S. (2014). *Why Liberians thought ebola was a government scam to attract Western aid.* Retrieved from http://www.thenation.com/article/why-liberians-thought-ebola-was-government-scam-attract-western-aid/

Jones, J. (2011). Ebola emerging: The limitations of culturalist discourses in epidemiology. *The Journal of Global Health, 1*(1), 4. Retrieved from http://www.ghjournal.org/ebola-emerging-the-limitations-of-culturalist-discourses-in-epidemiology/

Lamontagne, F., Clément, C., Fletcher, T., Jacob, S. T., Fischer, W. A., & Robert A. Fowler, R. A. (2014). Doing today's work superbly well: Treating ebola with current tools. *New England Journal of Medicine, 371, 1565-1566.* doi:10.1056/NEJMp1411310

Lazarus, R. S., & Folkman, S. (1984). *Stress, appraisal, and coping*. New York

Leroy, E. M., Gonzalez, J. P. & Baize, S. (2011). *Ebola and Marburg hae-morrhagic fever viruses: major scientific advances, but a relatively minor public health threat for Africa*. Retrieved from http://www.sciencedirect.com/science/article/pii/S1198743X14613744

Leroy E. M., Kumulungui B., Pourrut X., Rouquet P., Hassanin A., Yaba P., Delicat

A., Paweska, J. T., Gonzalez, J. P., & Swanepoel R. (2005). *Fruit bats as reservoirs of ebola virus*. Retrieved from http://www.ncbi.nlm.nih.gov/pubmed/16319873

Liberia Institute of Statistics and Geo-Information Services. (2014). *National population and housing census: Preliminary results*. Retrieved from http://www.emansion.gov.lr/doc/census_2008provisionalresults.pdf

Lincoln, Y. S., & Guba, E. G. (1985). *Naturalistic Inquiry*. Newbury Park, CA: Sage Publications.

McMillan, J. H., & Schumacher, S. (2001). *Research in education: A conceptual introduction* (5th ed.). New York: Longman.

Merriam, S. B. (2009). *Qualitative research: A guide to design and implementation*. San Francisco, CA: Jossey Bass.

Miller, B., & Morris, R. G. (2014). Virtual peer effects in Social learning theory. *Crime & Delinquency*, 1-27. doi:10.1177/0011128714526499

Patton, M. Q. (2001). *Qualitative research and evaluation methods* (2nd edition). Thousand Oaks, CA: Sage Publications.

Polit, D. F., & Beck, C. T. (2012). *Resource manual for nursing research: Generating and assessing evidence for nursing practice* (9th edition.). Philadelphia: Wolters Kluwer Health, Lippincott Williams & Wilkins.

Roach, J. B., Yadrick, M.K., Johnson, J.T., Boudreaux, L.J., Forsythe III, W.A., & Billon, W. (2003). Using self-efficacy to predict weight loss among young adults. *Journal of the American Dietetic Association, 103 (10), 1357-1359*

Ryan, R. M., & Deci, E. L. (2000). Self-determination theory and the facilitation of intrinsic motivation, social development, and well-being. *American Psychologist*. Retrieved from https://home.ubalt.edu/tmitch/641/deci_ryan_2000.pdf

Stajkovic, A. D., & Luthans, F. (1998b). Social cognitive theory and self-efficacy: Going beyond traditional motivational and behavioral approaches. *Organizational Dynamics, 76(4), 62-74*

Streubert, H. J., & Carpenter, D. R. (2011). *Qualitative research in nursing: advancing the humanistic imperative.* 5th ed. Philadelphia: Wolters Kluwer Health/Lippincott Williams & Wilkins.

Tambo, E. (2014). Non-conventional humanitarian interventions on ebola outbreak crisis in West Africa: Health, ethics and legal implications. *Journal of Infectious Diseases of Poverty, 2014; 3*: 42 doi:10.1186/2049-9957-3-42

Tosh, P. K., & Sampathkumar, P. (2014). What clinicians should know about the 2014 ebola outbreak. *Mayo Clinic Proceedings, 89(12), 1710-1717.* doi: 10.1016/j.mayocp.2014.10.010

Trochim, W. (2006). Research methods knowledge base. *Qualitative validity. 138* Retrieved from http://www.socialresearchmethods.net/kb/qualval.php

Usher K, & Grigg M. (2011). Responding to traumatic events. *Australian Nursing Journal, 18(9), 32-35.* Retrieved from http://e-publications.une.edu.au/1959.11/14669

World Health Organization. (2015). *Factors that contributed to the undetected spread of the Ebola virus and impeded rapid containment.* Retrieved from http://www.who.int/csr/disease/ebola/one-year-report/factors/en/

World Health Organization. (2014). *Ebola virus disease.* Retrieved from http://www.who.int/mediacentre/factsheets/fs103/en/

Yazan, B. (2015). Three approaches to case study methods in education: Yin, Merriam, and Stake. *The Qualitative Report, 20, 134-152.* Retrieved from http://www.nova.QR/QR20/2/yazan.pdf

Yin, R. K. (2011). *Qualitative research from start to finish.* New York: SAGE.

Yin, R. K. (2014). *Case study research: Design and methods.* Los Angeles: SAGE.

APPENDIX A

RESEARCH QUESTIONNAIRE
This study was designed to explore how residents of Monrovia coped with the threat of the 2014 Ebola virus disease (EVD) outbreak. The information collected from this study helped the researcher to understand the experiences of EVD survivors and their family caregivers. The researcher also solicited inputs from government officials, nongovernmental organizations staff, academicians, and reporters. Data for this study was collected through in-depth face-to-face interviews with 30 selected participants at a comfortable time and location. The purpose of this study was to explore the social, economic, and policy factors that contributed to the spread of the 2014 EVD outbreak in Liberia through a one-to-one interview process of participants. The research questionnaires for this study was developed by the researcher and pilot tested by at least two experts for relevance and alignment before conducting the study. The questions focus on factors that influenced the spread of the 2014 EVD and the experiences of survivors and their family caregivers who experience the phenomenon. Below are two categories of interview questions designed to answer the research goal:

INTERVIEW QUESTIONS 1 (EVD SURVIVORS OR FAMILY CAREGIVER)
1. How did you feel when you got diagnosed of having EVD?
2. How did your family members or friends react to the news upon hearing that you were diagnosed of EVD?
3. What do you think influence the spread of EVD?
4. How did government or NGO respond when you began to experience symptoms of EVD?
5. How did government response intended to contain the spread of EVD impact your cultural and traditional beliefs?

6. What is your reaction to government mandatory cremation and banning of public gatherings aimed at containing the spread of EVD?
7. What is life like being isolated in a barricaded tent and seeing people dressed in space-like-suits coming to treat you and how were you medically treated?
8. How did you feel when you heard that your relative was diagnosed of EVD?
9. How did you respond to your relative after seeing them suffering from EVD?
10. How did the media help you during the outbreak of EVD?
11. In economic terms, how did EVD impact you?
12. How did you cope with living under the threat of EVD?
13. How the national and international organizations did help you?
14. What recommendations would you make to the government, health workers, and policy makers to help contain future EVD outbreak?
15. In general, what does EVD mean to you?

INTERVIEW QUESTIONS 2 (GOVERNMENT, NGO, MEDIA, ACADEMICIANS)

1. How will you describe EVD and how did it impact you?
2. As (government official, NGO staff, a reporter from the media, or an academician), what was your role in helping to contain the spread of EVD?
3. How did government response such as mandatory cremation and banning of public gatherings intended to contain the spread of EVD impact residents of Monrovia?
4. What type of treatment did EVD patients received during isolation and did government or NGO have the capacity to treat EVD?
5. What do you think influence the spread of EVD?
6. How were EVD patients identified and transported to isolation tents?
7. How did media reporting help to educate communities about EVD?
8. As a reporter from the media, what access did you have to EVD patients, family caregivers, or their service providers?
9. As NGO, what was the working relationship between you and government?
10. In economic terms, how did EVD impact your work and the nation as a whole?
11. What recommendations would you make to government and global partners to help contain future EVD outbreak?

INTERVIEW SCRIPT

Before conducting the interview, an interview guide was developed to direct the conversation to the research topic and issues relating to the study. The interview guide was well scripted to meet the goal of the study. Throughout the interviews process, the researcher stated a script before commencing with the interview process as follows:

Thanks for accepting my invitation to participate in this interview today. My name is Augustine Manneh Sumo, and I am a researcher and Ph.D. student in Public Policy and Administration at the Walden University. I would want to understand your experience with the 2014 EVD outbreak. I will be asking you questions relating to the recent Ebola outbreak, and I will appreciate you provide me with answers best to your ability or knowledge. The purpose for this interview is to understand what it is like to cope with living under the threat of EVD. Please know that you can skip or decline to answer any question you fell you don't want to answer or you can stop this interview at any time if you no longer feel comfortable to participate. If you wish to receive a copy of the interview script, please feel free to ask for one. If you have any question regarding this interview, feel free to ask such question. Please know also that information gathered from this interview is strictly confidential and will not be shared with anyone other than the purpose for which it is obtained. By participating, you agree that you fully understand the terms and conditions of this interview. Generally, this study complied with the standard form produced by the Walden University. This study was designed to conduct a 45 minute to one hour face-to-face in-depth interview with each participant at their convenient time and location.

INFORMED CONSENT FORM

The approval by the IRB was first required before commencing the study. Secondly, research participants granted the researcher permission (consent) to be interviewed by reading and understanding the terms and conditions of the Walden's IRB Consent Form. The consent form was filled in by the researcher and explained in detail to the participant. Each participant read the form or they were read to, and confirmed that all parts of the form was well understood; the form was then signed and dated by both the researcher and the research participant. This process officially invited the research participant to participate in the study.

The purpose of the study was explained to the potential participants. The participants were told why they have been selected and the risks and benefits of the study were explained. Participants were also told of their rights such as to discontinue the interview at any time during the interview process if for whatever reason they become uncomfortable during the interview. The informed consent form according to Walden University standard was intended to minimize risk. This study obtained and documented all aspects of the informed consent form throughout the study.

APPENDIX B

COPING WITH THE THREAT OF EBOLA IN MONROVIA: A CASE STUDY
AUGUSTINE M. SUMO, TEL: 302 525 9453 EMAIL: AUGUSTINE.SUMO@WALDENU.EDU

You are invited to take part in a research study about Coping with the Threat of Ebola in Monrovia. This study will rely on the inputs from Ebola Virus Disease (EVD) survivors, their family caregivers, and officials of government, NGO staff, academicians, and reporters from the media who directly or indirectly experience EVD. This study is intended to understand how poverty and culture lifestyles influenced the spread of the 2014 EVD outbreak.

The researcher is inviting adult EVD survivor/family caregiver/official of government/NGO staff/academician/reporters from the media to be in the study. I obtained your name and contact information via the Ministry of Health and Social Welfare/Medicine Sans Frontier/Liberia National Red Cross. This form is part of a process called "informed consent" to allow you to understand this study before deciding whether to take part. This study is being conducted by a researcher named Augustine Manneh Sumo, who is a doctoral student at Walden University. My Walden University IRB approval number is 10-04-16-0166341 which expires on October 3, 2017.

BACKGROUND INFORMATION:

The purpose of this study is to explore how residents of Monrovia experience the phenomenon of coping with the threat of EVD. The study will explore the social, economic and policy factors that contributed to the spread of the

2014 EVD outbreak in Liberia. It is intended to investigate how mandatory cremation and government's regulations intended to contain the virus further contributed to the spread of EVD. It will explore how Monrovians perceive it and what their reactions were towards persons affected by EVD. It will also explain the public's perception and change in attitudes and the meanings they ascribe to EVD.

PROCEDURES:

If you agree to be in this study, you will be asked to:

- voluntarily participate in one or two interviews
- that each interview could last between 45 minutes to one hour
- that each interview will be taped recorded
- not present any personal identifier during the interview, to ensure your anonymity
- participants must be 18 years old or above
- participants must be an EVD survivor, family caregiver who lived in Monrovia during the 2014 EVD outbreak
- participants must be a reporter from the media who covered the event
- participants must be an official of government or NGO staff who provided care and services to EVD survivors
- participants must be willing to participate in the interview process without any monetary compensation

Here are some sample questions:
- How did you feel when you got diagnosed of having EVD?
- How did your family members or friends react to the news upon hearing that you were diagnosed of EVD?
- What do you think influence the spread of EVD?
- How will you describe EVD and how did it impact you?
- As (government official, NGO staff, a reporter from the media, or an academician), what was your role in helping to contain the spread of EVD?

VOLUNTARY NATURE OF THE STUDY:

This study is voluntary. You are free to accept or turn down the invitation. You can also decide not to answer any question you feel uncomfortable during the interview. No one at the Ministry of Health/Medicine Sans Frontier/Liberia National Red Cross will treat you differently if you decide not to be in the study. If you decide to be in the study now, you can still change your mind later. You may stop at any time. Your contact information will be retained only for the purpose of sharing the results and will not be associated with the interview data.

RISKS AND BENEFITS OF BEING IN THE STUDY:

Being in this type of study involves some risk of the minor discomforts that can be encountered in daily life, such as a reminder of your past experience (emotion) or stress. Being in this study would not pose risk to your safety or wellbeing. It is hoped that the results of this study will benefit the community through providing greater insight into finding a controlled mechanism and or cure for Ebola.

PAYMENT:

Participation in this study is voluntary and will involve no costs or payments to you.

PRIVACY:

Reports coming out of this study will not share the identities of individual participants. All information collected during the study period will be kept strictly confidential. Details that might identify participants, such as the location of the study, also will not be shared. The researcher will not use your personal information for any purpose outside of this research project. Data will be kept secure by a password protected computer, locked cabinet and codes will be used in place of names. Data will be kept for a period of at least 5 years, as required by the university.

CONTACTS AND QUESTIONS:

You may ask any questions you have now. Or if you have questions later, you may contact the researcher via telephone number 302 525 9453 or by email at augustine.sumo@waldenu.edu. If you want to talk privately about your rights as a participant, you can call the Research Participant Advocate at my university at +1 612-312-1210, email at: irb@waldenu.edu. The researcher will give you a copy of this consent form to keep.

Obtaining Your Consent:

If you feel you understand the study well enough to make a decision about it, please indicate your consent by signing below.

Name of Participant	
Date of Consent	
Participant's Signature	
Researcher's Signature	

APPENDIX C

DATE_____________

COPING WITH THE THREAT OF EBOLA IN MONROVIA: A CASE STUDY

READ: LETTER OF INVITATION TO PARTICIPATE IN RESEARCH STUDY

Dear ___,

My name is Augustine Manneh Sumo. I am a student in the Public Policy and Administration Department at the Walden University. I am conducting a research study as part of the requirements for my degree in Doctor of Philosophy Public Policy and Administration – Law and Public Policy, and I would like to invite you to participate in the study.

I am studying to explore the social, economic and policy factors that contributed to the spread of the 2014 Ebola Virus Disease (EVD) outbreak in Liberia. This study will rely on inputs from you to understand how poverty and culture lifestyles may have influenced the spread of the 2014 EVD outbreak in Monrovia. If you decide to participate, you will be given a call by me to arrange a meeting where we can discuss the detail of the study.

Upon discussing and understanding the purpose of the study, I will ask if you would like to participate in the study. And if you agree to participate, an Informed Consent Form will be signed by you to authorize your participation. An initial interview date will then be scheduled. The interview will take place at a location convenience to you. In particular, we will discuss Coping with the Threat of Ebola in Monrovia. The interview will be audiotaped and notes taken so that I can accurately reflect on what is discussed. The tapes will only be reviewed by me the researcher who will transcribe and analyze it. The tape recording will then be destroyed.

You can decline to answer any question or leave the interview in case you may feel uncomfortable answering some of the questions. You do not have to answer any questions that you do not wish to. Although you probably won't benefit directly from participating in this study, we hope that others in the community or society, in general, will benefit by providing greater insight into finding a controlled mechanism and or cure for Ebola.

Participation is confidential. Study information will be kept in a secure location during the study. The results of the study may be published or presented at professional meetings, but your identity will not be revealed. In other words, participation is anonymous, which means that no one will know what your answers are.

I will be happy to answer any questions you have about the study. You may contact me at 0880 511 561/+1302 525 9453 or augustine.sumo@waldenu.edu if you have study related questions or problems.

Thank you for your consideration. If you would like to participate, please give me a call or email me at the above contact information. Otherwise, I will be making a follow-up contact with you within the next few days to see whether you are willing to participate.

With kind regards,

Augustine Manneh Sumo
Tel: +1 302 525 9453
Email: augustine.sumo@waldenu.edu

APPENDIX D

COPING WITH THE THREAT OF EBOLA IN MONROVIA: A CASE STUDY

(One page for each research participant)

Interview Protocol Title:

Date: _______________________________ Time: _______________________________

Location: ____

Interviewer: ____

Interviewee(s): ____(code name)

Opening statement/brief description of project: [READ] Includes: Investigator motive; purpose of study; protection of respondents, including confidentiality, willingness to continue participation, use of data, access to final report, and permission to record interview.

Grand tour question:
A. Probes (if used, depending how structured the interview)
B. [RESEARCHER THOUGHTS BRACKETED]

Sub-questions:
A. Probes (if used, depending how structured the interview)
B. [RESEARCHER THOUGHTS BRACKETED]

[Thank participants]

APPENDIX E

COPING WITH THE THREAT OF EBOLA IN MONROVIA: A CASE STUDY
OBSERVATIONAL PROTOCOL

Direct observations – In addition to information gathered during interviews, participants will also be observed. Each meeting or interview time will vary between 45 minutes to one hour. During this time of observation, an observation data collection form (enclosed below) will be used to record field notes and research reflections.

Participants – Potential participants will include Ebola survivors and their family caregivers, officials of government from the Ministry of Health and Social Welfare of Liberia, NGO staff from the Liberia National Red Cross, and Médecins Sans Frontières. Other participants will include academicians and members of the media. I intend to spend time observing these participants during interviews or meetings. This will involve observing and taking notes to describe activities, interactions and discourses relating to the impact of Ebola on individuals and the community as a whole.

Consent Process – Data collection will only begin after the IRB approval. I am required to seek written informed consent from each participant that will participate in the study in advance of observations and interviews. The nature and purpose of the research will be explained and participants will be free to withdraw from being observed at any time during the case study.

Observation Procedures – This case study observation will require that I follow the activities of those being studied through interactions. I will attempt to capture in field notes a detailed description of activities relating to their activities or behaviors. I will attempt to explain and interpret the behavior of each participant. I will principally be observing activities and interactions, but will also ask questions for clarification and will ask individual participants about their experiences, seeking to bring to light logics, concerns, and meanings that emerge from the observational activities.

Generally - Discussions and interviews will be recorded manually in field notes, to provide more detailed information. I intend to digitally record informal interviews or discussions for later transcription. From these observations, I will attempt to produce a thick description of the impact of the 2014 Ebola outbreak in Monrovia. Below is a summary of my proposed observational protocol.

Date: ______________________________Time: ______________________________

Length of activity: ____(minutes)

Site: ____

Participants:____

Grand tour question: (Questions will be based on participants' behavior – see interview questions)

Descriptive Notes:

Physical Setting:

____

____

____

____

____

Description of individuals engaged in activity:

____

____

____

____

____

Sequence of activity over time:

____

____

____

____

____

____

Interactions:

____

____

____

____

____

____

Unplanned events:

____

____

____

____

____

Participants comments: (expressed in quotes)

____

____

____

____

____

____

Reflective comments: (questions to self, observations of nonverbal behavior, my interpretations)

____

____

____

____

____

____

My observation of what seemed to occurred:

____

____

____

____

____

____